Non-Orthopedic EMERGENCY CARE in Athletics

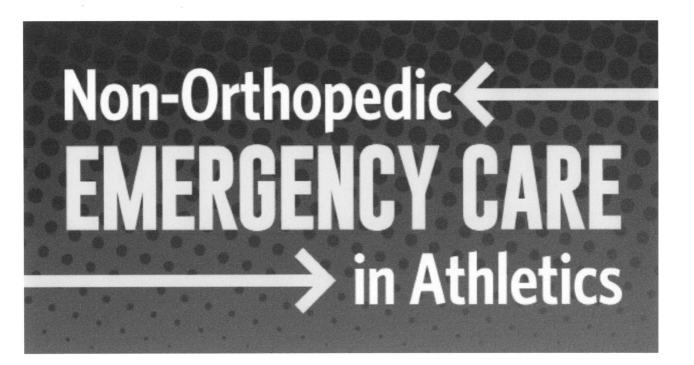

Non-Orthopedic EMERGENCY CARE in Athletics

Francis Feld, DNP, CRNA, LAT, ATC, NRP
UPMC Passavant Hospital Staff CRNA
Prehospital RN Ross West View EMSA
Medical Group Supervisor, Allegheny County Hazmat Medical Team
Pittsburgh, Pennsylvania

Keith M. Gorse, EdD, LAT, ATC
Assistant Professor and Clinical Coordinator
Department of Athletic Training
Duquesne University
Pittsburgh, Pennsylvania

Robert O. Blanc, MS, LAT, ATC, EMT-P
Head Athletic Trainer—Football
Adjunct Clinical Instructor
University of Pittsburgh, ATEP
Pittsburgh, Pennsylvania

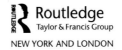
Routledge
Taylor & Francis Group

NEW YORK AND LONDON

First published in 2020 by SLACK Incorporated

Published 2024 by Routledge
605 Third Avenue, New York, NY 10158

and by Routledge
4 Park Square, Milton Park, Abingdon, Oxon OX14 4RN

Routledge is an imprint of the Taylor & Francis Group, an informa business

Cover Artist: Katherine Christie

Library of Congress Cataloging-in-Publication Data

Names: Feld, Francis, 1954- editor. | Gorse, Keith M., editor. | Blanc,
    Robert O., 1960- editor.
Title: Nonorthopedic emergency care in athletics / [edited by] Francis
    Feld, Keith M. Gorse, Robert O. Blanc.
Description: First edition. | Thorofare, NJ : SLACK Incorporated, [2020] |
    Includes bibliographical references and index.
Identifiers: LCCN 2019038353 | ISBN 9781630916176 (paperback)
Subjects: MESH: Emergency Treatment | Sports | First Aid | Emergency
    Medical Services | Athletic Injuries | Emergencies
Classification: LCC RA645.5 | NLM WA 292 | DDC 362.18--dc23
LC record available at https://lccn.loc.gov/2019038353

ISBN: 9781630916176 (pbk)
ISBN: 9781003525196 (ebk)

DOI: 10.4324/9781003525196

DEDICATION

To all the health care providers who are devoted to the development and implementation of proper emergency care for people who are involved at the recreational, high school, college, and professional levels of athletics.

CONTENTS

ACKNOWLEDGMENTS

Many people have assisted us during the year that *Non-Orthopedic Emergency Care in Athletics* has been in production. The staff at SLACK Incorporated was both supportive and patient during the entire process of developing this textbook. In particular, we thank Mr. Brien Cummings, who provided the continuing support that gave us the initial okay to proceed and help make the book happen. We also thank all our contributors for their efforts in helping put together this textbook.

Francis Feld thanks the contributors for providing the material that makes this a unique textbook for athletic medicine professionals. Management of serious conditions requires education and experience, plus the wisdom to calmly apply them in a critical situation when others may be in a panic. This text supplies the education, but readers must develop the experience and wisdom necessary to perform well in a crisis. Francis also thanks his wife, Christine, for her love and support. Keith and Rob deserve special consideration for occasionally throwing out the sea anchor and keeping this ship from running aground during development.

Keith Gorse thanks both Fran and Rob for their mentorship, guidance, and friendship over the last 30-plus years. Keith also thanks his wonderful family (Betsy, Erin, and Tyler) for their never-ending support through all his years as an athletic trainer, a husband, and a father. Without them, his professional career and personal life would not have a whole lot of meaning.

Robert Blanc thanks everyone involved in the writing of this material, especially Keith and Fran, who have taken the lead in providing our profession, as well as others, with the most comprehensive information necessary for the excellent care of active individuals. Keith and Fran have led the way with their professionalism and dedication to making athletic training better for all. Rob also thanks his wife, Peggy, for unmatched patience and support throughout the years.

CONTRIBUTING AUTHORS

Joseph Andrie, MD (Chapter 3)
UPMC St. Margaret
Pittsburgh, Pennsylvania

Christian Conte, PhD (Chapter 11)
Emotional Management
Pittsburgh, Pennsylvania

Donald J. Conte, MS, MA (Chapter 11)
Professor Emeritus
California University of Pennsylvania
California, Pennsylvania

Harsh K. Desai, MD (Chapter 12)
UPMC Passavant Hospital
Pittsburgh, Pennsylvania

Jason Ferderber, MD (Chapter 4)
UPMC Department of Emergency Medicine
Pittsburgh, Pennsylvania

Kevin Garrett, MD (Chapter 12)
Chief of Surgery
UPMC Passavant Hospital
Pittsburgh, Pennsylvania

Kelley Henderson, EdD, LAT, ATC (Chapter 13)
Nova Southeastern University
Fort Lauderdale, Florida

Shane Hennessy, DO (Chapter 7)
UPMC Sports Medicine
Pittsburgh, Pennsylvania

Christine M. Leeper, MD (Chapter 12)
Chief Resident
UPMC General Surgery
Pittsburgh, Pennsylvania

Sarah Manspeaker, PhD, LAT, ATC (Chapter 13)
Duquesne University
Pittsburgh, Pennsylvania

Aaron V. Mares, MD (Chapter 7)
UPMC and Team Physician
University of Pittsburgh Football Team
Pittsburgh, Pennsylvania

Ryan P. McGovern, PhD, LAT, ATC (Chapter 10)
Texas Health Sports Medicine
Allen, Texas

James Medure (Chapter 5)
University of Pittsburgh Football Team
Pittsburgh, Pennsylvania

Vincent Mosesso Jr, MD (Chapter 4)
UPMC Emergency Medicine
Pittsburgh, Pennsylvania

John Murphy, DO (Chapter 5)
UPMC Sports Medicine
Pittsburgh, Pennsylvania

John Panos, MEd, LAT, ATC, EMT (Chapter 3)
Fox Chapel High School
Pittsburgh, Pennsylvania

Timothy Rausch, MSN, CRNP (Chapter 8)
Nurse Practitioner
AGH Trauma
Pittsburgh, Pennsylvania

Matthew Schaffer, MD (Chapter 3)
UPMC and Team Physician
Fox Chapel High School
Pittsburgh, Pennsylvania

Alan Shapiro, DO (Chapter 9)
UPMC Passavant Hospital
Pittsburgh, Pennsylvania

INTRODUCTION

Keith, Rob, and I have been friends and colleagues for more than 30 years, and while our careers have developed differently, we have always believed that the athletic trainer is the foundation of any athletic medicine program. As the gatekeeper, the athletic trainer must have a working knowledge of virtually any medical problem that may arise with athletes and how to seek appropriate and timely care. Emergency care textbooks for the athletic population have uniformly focused on head, neck, and orthopedic problems, with scant focus on the much larger topic of medical conditions that may arise in a youthful population; though not seen commonly, they can be deadly if unrecognized and untreated. There is also a subset of health care providers other than athletic trainers, especially at the youth sports level, who find themselves providing initial medical care at athletic events because of family involvement.

We have assembled an interprofessional group of health care providers who have covered what we feel are the most crucial types of serious medical emergencies that may be encountered in sports. We hope this text provides information that is helpful to all who provide care for athletes at any level and in any sport.

It should be emphasized that some of the interventions described in this text may not be within the scope of practice for all health care providers, and readers must consult their individual state practice laws to determine what is and what is not appropriate for their practice.

—*Francis Feld, DNP, CRNA, LAT, ATC, NRP*

1

Design and Implementation of Emergency Action Plans and Standard Operating Procedures

Keith M. Gorse, EdD, LAT, ATC

Chapter Key Words

- Emergency action plan
- Emergency team personnel
- Pregame and pre-event medical time out
- Standard operating procedures
- Specific venue locations

Chapter Scenario

A jury in a Court of Common Pleas awarded a 14-year-old $1.7 million in damages against 2 local youth baseball athletic associations.

The youth male baseball player, then age 11, was hit by a foul ball while in the dugout during a game played at the community park baseball field. The boy was badly injured, and medical testimony was presented that there would be long-term consequences, as well as pain and suffering, from the injury.

The attorney for the boy said that the defendants were responsible for the injury because the dugout was not properly protected by a fence to prevent foul balls from entering that area. There was evidence that such fences are required by the Little League's emergency action plans (EAPs) and standard operating procedures (SOPs) and are customary at all Little League Inc. baseball fields.

Right after the incident, the father took his son to a local hospital, and the boy was then rushed to Children's

Hospital, where he underwent brain surgery. As a result of his injuries, the player sustained a fractured skull, brain shift, and bleeding on his brain, as well as severe changes in behavior, mood, and impulse control.

"He woke up a different person," his father said. "His whole personality changed."

The boy changed schools and now is accompanied by special education teachers in his classes. According to his father, he has struggled with his studies and has pain every day.

During research into the lawsuit, investigators discovered that another child, who was in the same dugout, had been struck in the chest by a foul ball 1 year earlier. However, the child was wearing a chest protector and was not injured.

"They knew it, and nobody did anything," the boy's father said. "They let it go."

According to Little League Inc. safety policies, all dugouts need to be fenced and screened, and the attorney indicated that the dugout at this particular baseball field did not meet the organization's standards.

Scenario Resolution

One week after the young player's injury, the rest of the fencing was added to the dugout, and 1 month after that, venue-specific EAPs with SOPs were developed and approved by the local township parks and recreation department and the youth baseball league.

Feld F., Gorse KM, Blanc RO
Non-Orthopedic Emergency Care in Athletics (pp 1-8).
© 2020 Taylor & Francis Group.

INTRODUCTION

Emergency medical situations may occur in athletics at any given time. When they do, it is important to have the proper EAPs with SOPs in place to provide the best possible care to athletes with possible life-threatening injuries or illness. The design and implementation of the EAP will help ensure that the quality of care provided to the athletes is the best possible. The goal of the sports medicine staff of any athletic organization (eg, academic, amateur, and professional) is that the EAP will minimize the time needed to provide an immediate response to a potentially life-threatening situation or medical emergency.

Because medical emergencies can occur during any practice and/or event, the sports medicine staff must be prepared for any situation. Emergency care preparation includes the formation of a venue-specific EAP, proper coverage of athletic events and practices, maintenance of emergency equipment, use of appropriate personnel involved with the medical emergency, efficient communication with proper directions, and the continuing education and practice of emergency medical care staff. Even if the athletic organization and its sports medicine staff have taken every precaution to prevent occurrences, medical emergencies may still happen. With proper organization, education, and practice, the emergency personnel can manage most athletic medical emergency situations in a timely, effective, and professional manner.

The organization and administration of emergency care in athletic activities includes the following components:
- design and implementation,
- legal need and duty,
- emergency team personnel,
- emergency equipment,
- emergency communication,
- specific venue locations,
- emergency transportation,
- emergency care facilities, and
- pregame and pre-event medical time out.

This chapter provides an agenda for emergency care involving athletic trainers and other health care providers from an organizational perspective. The major topics will concern issues relating to the development and contents of EAPs and SOPs. The chapter will also explain the legal need for emergency planning and the proper documentation to reduce the liability factor and, therefore, the chances of a lawsuit.

Design and Implementation

Over the past 2 decades, many research projects involving athletics at all levels found that almost one-third of athletes competing were injured in a way that required medical attention.[1] The National Athletic Trainers' Association (NATA) position statement recommends that each organization and/or institution sponsoring athletic activities and events should design and implement a written emergency plan.[2] The EAPs and SOPs need to be designed with the help of organizational and/or institutional personnel in consultation with local emergency medical services (EMS) and emergency care facilities.

The EAP needs to be implemented for the safety of all athletic personnel, including athletes, coaches, and officials. It should be concise, yet detailed enough to facilitate prompt and appropriate action. The development of an EAP and proper use of this plan can often make the difference in the outcome of an injury situation. All components of an EAP are connected, and they must all be considered to ensure a complete and favorable outcome in a potentially dangerous situation. When the importance of the EAP is realized and the plan has been designed, it must be implemented through documentation of the plan, education of those involved, and frequent rehearsal of the plan itself.[2]

The EAP must provide a clear explanation of how it is going to work, allowing continuity among all members of the athletic training staff and other emergency team personnel. It is important to have a separate plan for different athletic venues and for practices versus games. Emergency medical team personnel, such as team physicians, may not be present at all athletic events, and this should be considered during development of the EAP. In addition, the specific location and type of equipment required may vary among the sports teams and venues. For example, outdoor sports with a high risk of heat illness exposure may require a large tub or wading pool for emergency cooling of athletes at risk of heat stroke. This equipment would not be required for indoor sports.

It is important to educate all medical team personnel regarding the EAP and its contents. All team personnel should be familiar with the EMS that provide coverage to the venues. Each emergency team member, as well as the athletic organization administrators, should have a written copy of the EAP that provides complete documentation of their roles and responsibilities in all emergency situations. Copies of the EAP specific to each venue should be posted by a prominent marked position at that venue.[2]

All members of the medical team need to practice the EAP. This provides the team members with a chance to maintain their emergency skills at a high level of competency. It also provides the opportunity for athletic trainers and other emergency personnel to communicate regarding specific procedures in their respective areas. The EAP rehearsal can be accomplished via meetings held several times throughout the year. One suggestion is to rehearse prior to the preseason for high-risk sports such as football in the fall, ice hockey in the winter, and lacrosse in the spring. Updates should be addressed as needed throughout the year, as venues, emergency medical procedures, and emergency team personnel may change at any time.

Legal Need and Duty

There is a legal need and duty for emergency team personnel to develop EAPs to ensure that the highest quality of care is provided to all physically active sports participants. The emergency team, including athletic trainers, is measured in part by the standards of care provided to athletes, which is 1 reason it is important to have a written document.[3,4] The NATA has indicated that a well-organized and well-written EAP document that is regularly rehearsed is essential for all athletic organizations and sports medicine programs.[2,5,6]

The athletic organization administrators and emergency medical team personnel must anticipate that a possible medical situation may occur during any athletic activity. Injuries to the head, spine, and limbs are possible in both practice and competition. A duty exists on the part of the athletic organization and the emergency team to provide proper care for any medical conditions that result from athletic participation. Although it is not common in athletic activity, the athletic trainers and the rest of the emergency team must always be prepared for any type of life- or limb-threatening injury. Failure to have an EAP in place and to rehearse it regularly may result in inefficient or inadequate care, which could lead to charges of negligence against the athletic organization administration and emergency team personnel.[2,7]

Several legal cases have supported the need for written EAPs. The most prominent is *Kleinknecht vs Gettysburg College,* which went to court in 1993.[8] As part of the decision, the Court stated that Gettysburg College owed a duty to all recruited athletes and that the college must provide "prompt and adequate emergency services while athletes were engaged in school-sponsored intercollegiate athletic activities."[8] The same court also ruled that reasonable measures must be ensured and in place to provide adequate and prompt treatment in any emergency situation.[8] It can be concluded from this ruling that planning is critical to ensure that athletes receive proper emergency care, which further reinforces the need for a written EAP as a requirement for all athletic organizations.[2,8]

It is also important to involve athletic organization administrators, sport coaches, and sports medicine staff in the development process of the EAP (Figure 1-1). The EAP needs to be updated annually by all involved emergency team personnel. All revisions to the EAP must be approved by members at all levels of the athletic organization, as well as emergency team members, including local EMS.[7]

Emergency Team Personnel

The implementation of an EAP cannot take place without the formation of an emergency team. The emergency team personnel consists of members of the sports medicine staff, including the certified athletic trainer and the team physician. The sports medicine staff is responsible for the formation of the EAP for the entire athletic organization.[9] When a potential situation occurs, the emergency team can vary depending on who is at the scene. The emergency team can include certified athletic trainers, team physicians, local EMS, athletic training students, team coaches, equipment managers, and school nurses. Any member of the emergency team can act as a first responder—a person who has been trained to provide emergency care before EMS personnel arrives on scene.[2,10]

All personnel within the emergency team should be required to be certified in cardiopulmonary resuscitation (CPR), automatic external defibrillation (AED), and prevention of disease transmission (eg, Occupational Safety and Health Administration blood-borne pathogens). An extensive EAP review should be required for all emergency team personnel associated with athletic practices and all events and competitions.[11]

The roles of the personnel of the emergency team will vary depending on how many people are on the team, the specific venue being used, and the preferences of the certified athletic trainer, who is usually in charge of the design and implementation of the EAP. Roles of the team personnel should include immediate care of the athlete/patient, emergency equipment retrieval, communication to EMS, and proper transport to the emergency care facility.[9]

When assembling the emergency team, it is important to allow each member of the team to adapt to all emergency role situations that may occur. It may be a good idea to have more than 1 individual assigned to each of the designated roles. This allows the emergency team to function without delay in an event where some personnel may not always be present.

Emergency Equipment

All appropriate emergency equipment and supplies must be on hand at all athletic practices and events. All assigned emergency team personnel should be aware of the location and function of all emergency equipment and supplies. Ensure that all emergency equipment can be properly inventoried and maintained on an annual basis and stored in a secure storage area for safekeeping by the athletic training staff.[12]

All school and organization members must recognize the importance of the availability of AEDs (Figure 1-2) as indicated by guidelines set forth by the American Heart Association and the National Safety Council.[11,13] These guidelines indicate that early defibrillation is considered a critical component of basic life support. It is also important to use proper airway techniques for resuscitation when necessary. Emergency team personnel should be educated in the proper use of AEDs and airway adjuncts before being allowed to use them.[14,15]

All emergency equipment must be in good operating condition and should be checked on a regular basis. An emergency situation is not the time to find out that a piece

ROBERT MORRIS UNIVERSITY NEVILLE ISLAND SPORTS COMPLEX
Components of the Emergency Action Plan
and Standard Operating Procedure
Authorization Form

1. Emergency Personnel: Athletic Trainers – EMS – Police and Fire – Coaches

2. Emergency Communication: Permanent Phone Locations
                             Emergency Phone Numbers
                             Communication Trees

3. Emergency Equipment: First Aid Supplies – AEDs – Splints – Spine Boards

4. Emergency Education: CPR/First Aid & AED – Coaches Palm Cards

5. Emergency Mapping: Venue Maps – Diagrams and Written Directions
                       Hospital Emergency Room Locations and Directions

The importance of being properly prepared when athletic emergencies arise cannot be stressed enough. A student athlete's survival may hinge on how trained and prepared athletic department staff is in acting and communicating in a medical emergency. It is also important on how fast emergency personnel react and travel to the athletic venues in case of an accident. It is prudent to invest in athletic department "ownership" in the emergency plan by involving the athletic administration – coaches – athletic trainers and team physicians. It is also important to educate all athletic department personnel in CPR-AED – First Aid training and to know all emergency phone numbers. Through development and implementation of the emergency plan, the athletic training department helps ensure that the student athlete will have the best care provided if an emergency situation arises.

Approved:

_____ Athletic Trainer   Date: _____

_____ Athletic Director   Date: _____

_____ Team Physician   Date: _____

_____ Risk Managment   Date: _____

_____ General Mgr, ISC   Date: _____

Figure 1-1. EAP / SOP legal authorization form. (Source: Robert Morris University. Athletics Emergency Action Plan and Standard Operating Procedures for 2017-18. Athletic Training Handbook. 2017.)

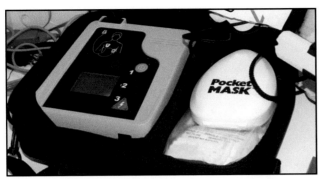

Figure 1-2. Game/event sideline emergency AED equipment.

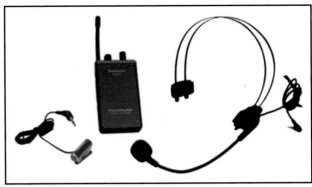

Figure 1-3. Communication gear used for athletic events.

of emergency equipment is missing or is not working. Each emergency team member must be trained in advance on how to use all first aid equipment and supplies. Finally, all emergency team personnel should regularly practice with all safety equipment so there is no delay in the effective use of the equipment during an actual emergency.

Emergency Communication

Proper communication setup is the key to quick and effective delivery of acute care in any emergency trauma situation. Athletic trainers and all other emergency team personnel, including EMS, must work together to provide the best possible care for injured athletes. Communication prior, during, and after an event is a good way to establish a positive working relationship among all groups of professionals.[16,17] If emergency medical transportation is not available on site at a specific venue during a practice or event, then direct communication with the EMS at the time of injury or illness will be necessary.

Access to any working telecommunications device, whether fixed (landline) or mobile, should be mandatory. The emergency communications system needs to be checked and put into service by all personnel prior to each practice and event to ensure it is in proper working order.[10,18] A secondary back-up communications plan should be created in case the primary emergency communication system fails. Currently, the most common methods of communication are cellular telephones and handheld (mobile) radios (Figure 1-3). However, at any specific athletic venue, it is important to know the location of a working, fixed telephone, as cellular service may not always be reliable or the batteries in the cell phones and mobile radios may fail.

A list of all appropriate emergency phone and radio numbers, such as local EMS, should be posted by the communication system most used by the athletic trainers and be readily available to all emergency team personnel. Specific directions to on-site venues should also be included and posted with the emergency numbers. Such directions should include the actual street address of the venue, main road, secondary road, and other landmark information that

will assist EMS personnel in arriving at the scene as soon as possible.[19]

Specific Venue Locations

The EAP should be specific to venue locations and any additional features that could be part of the facility (Figure 1-4). The EAP for each venue should include information concerning the accessibility to emergency team personnel, communications systems, emergency equipment, and emergency vehicle transportation systems.[2,5]

At all home-specific venues, the host athletic trainer should communicate the EAP for the venue to the visiting team and its medical personnel. Specific areas reviewed should include all available emergency team personnel, location of communication systems, and available emergency equipment.

At neutral or away venues, the athletic trainer or any other member of the emergency team should identify the availability of communication details regarding EMS for that location.[2,5] It is also important that the name and location of the nearest emergency care facility and the availability of emergency transportation at the venue are identified prior to the event.

Emergency Transportation

The EAPs and SOPs should include a policy for transportation of the injured person for all athletic practices and events. By definition, an emergency dictates that transport to local health care facilities should be via a proper EMS ambulance vehicle. The policy on transportation should explain in detail when and where an ambulance is to be located during all athletic events.[1] Emphasis should be placed on having an ambulance on site for all high-risk or collision sporting events such as football, soccer, lacrosse, and ice hockey.[7] In some cases, the number of spectators who are expected to attend an event may warrant the presence of 1 or more ambulances, even if the sport is not considered a collision type or high risk. Although spectators typically are not the responsibility of the emergency team, this point should be made clear with the administrators. If

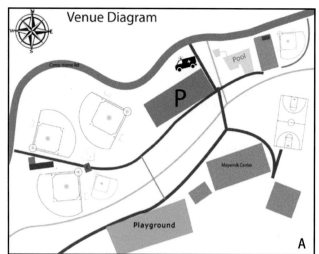

Figure 1-4. EAP diagram of athletic venue location.

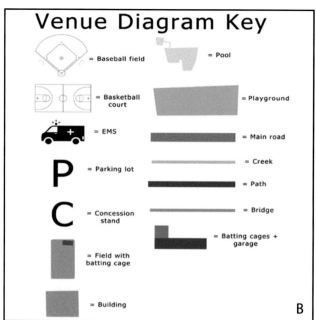

the team's medical staff is also responsible for the care of spectators, staffing for the event and the EAP itself must reflect this fact.

When developing a transportation policy, EMS response time to an accident should always be considered. Consideration should also be given to the level of transportation service and equipment that is available. An example of this would be that of basic life support versus advanced life support availability. Another issue that must be reviewed is the level of training of all emergency personnel who staff the attending ambulance service.[19,20]

It is critical that working emergency communication systems are in place between the on-site medical staff and the EMS that would be dispatching an ambulance in an emergency.[16] In the event that an ambulance is on site, a location should be designated for the ambulance with clear, direct access to the competition area and a clear route for entering and exiting the athletic venue.[19]

Emergency Care Facilities

The EAP should include information regarding the transportation directions to an emergency care facility from all athletic venues. When selecting an appropriate emergency care facility, consider the proximity of the emergency facility to the venues and the level of care available at the facility.[2]

Notify the emergency care facility and local EMS that are used by the athletic organization in advance of all athletic events that are scheduled at any of the organization's venues.[1] The EAP should be reviewed and practiced with both the emergency care facility administrators and emergency medical personnel regarding important information concerning athlete care. An example of the information

that must be reviewed is the proper removal of athletic equipment, such as football helmets and shoulder pads, at the local emergency care facility.[21]

Pregame and Pre-Event Medical Time Out

One of the best ways in which emergency team personnel and local EMS can collaborate with each other is by conducting a medical time out prior to most athletic games or events (Figure 1-5). The pregame or pre-event medical time out was introduced in 2012 by the NATA and was modeled from health care facility operating rooms conducting a surgical time out before a procedure to ensure correct patient care.[22]

The NATA initiative calls for all personnel of the emergency team to meet, ensuring that everyone is on the same page before a potentially life-threatening injury or situation occurs. In addition to reviewing the venue-specific EAPs and SOPs, the medical time out should also include discussion of the following event items[22]:

- Role and location of each emergency team personnel present.
- Communications plan, method, devices, and primary and secondary means of communicating.
- Location of local EMS personnel and ambulance.
- Proper transportation and directions to local health care facility if needed.
- Emergency equipment on site, at a known location.
- The presence of crowd control that may inhibit emergency care.
- Personnel questions or concerns.

When a life-threatening injury or situation occurs in an athletic competition, the response by emergency team

---

PREGAME MEDICAL TIME-OUT TEAM MEETING

(60-minute Pregame Meeting)
- *Led by head team physician for the home team*
- *Introduce each team member – name and role*
- *Head team physicians*
- *Head athletic trainers*
- *2 UNCs (specify team to be covered)*
- *2 ATC Spotters (specify team to be covered)*
- *1 AMP • 1 VTML*
- *Referee and alternate official*
- *Lead EMS person for stadium*
- *NFL Football Operations representative*
- *Verify stadium location of ambulance, transport cart, spine board, defibrillator, and advanced airway equipment*
- *Review location of stadium exit for emergent transport scenario*
- *Review EAP medical facility and other medical facilities that may be used*
- *Review location of x-ray equipment and technician*
- *Questions or concerns*

Figure 1-5. NFL pregame medical time-out meeting agenda. (Adapted from ATC Spotters. Another Set of Eyes for Injuries. NFL Football Operations. https://operations.nfl.com/the-game/gameday-behind-the-scenes/atc-spotters/. August, 2018. Accessed June 2, 2019.)

personnel and local EMS providers must be coordinated in a professional and proper manner. Developing professional relationships, using the venue-specific EAPs and SOPs, and using a proper medical time out prior to athletic games and events will help lead to the highest quality of emergency care.[19,22]

CHAPTER SUMMARY

- Organizations that sponsor athletic activities must have a written EAP with SOPs. The EAPs and SOPs should be able to be adapted to any emergency situation.
- The EAPs and SOPs must be written documents and should be distributed to all members of the emergency team. This includes certified athletic trainers, team physicians, athletic training students, EMS, coaches, and school nurses.
- All personnel involved with the organization and involved with the EAPs and SOPs share a professional and legal duty to provide the best emergency care to an injured individual. This includes the responsibility of developing and implementing an EAP and SOP.
- The athletic organization's EAPs and SOPs identify the personnel involved in carrying out the plan and outline their qualifications. All emergency team members

should be trained and certified in CPR, AED, first aid, and blood-borne pathogen prevention.
- The EAPs and SOPs should provide the personnel of the emergency team with information on initial patient assessment and care.
- The EAPs and SOPs should specify all equipment and supplies needed to help carry out the tasks required in case of an emergency. The plan should also outline the location of all emergency equipment.
- The EAPs and SOPs should establish a clear mechanism for communication with the appropriate EMS in the area. Identification of the type of transportation for the injured individual(s) should also be part of the plan.
- The EAPs and SOPs should be specific to each activity site and venue. Each site and venue should have a separate plan that is derived from the overall organizational policies on emergency planning.
- The EAPs and SOPs should incorporate the emergency care facilities, such as local hospital emergency departments, being used for the care of the injured individuals.
- Pre-event medical time outs should occur between all emergency team personnel and local EMS before every event, ensuring that everyone is on the same page before a potentially life-threatening injury occurs.

CHAPTER REVIEW QUESTIONS

1. The EAPs and SOPs should be specific to:
   a) each activity
   b) each venue location
   c) one specific site
   d) a and b only

2. The EAPs and SOPs should be reviewed and rehearsed by the emergency team:
   a) only once per year
   b) as many times as possible
   c) no more than twice per year
   d) 3 or 4 times per year

3. Professional responsibilities for emergency team members include:
   a) CPR training
   b) first aid training
   c) blood-borne pathogen training
   d) all of the above

4. When the EAPs and SOPs have been developed, they are implemented through:
   a) documentation
   b) education
   c) practice
   d) all of the above

5. Which of the following conditions should be reviewed during a pregame or pre-event medical time out between local EMS and emergency team personnel?
   a) suspected fractures
   b) injuries to the head or spine
   c) abdominal injuries
   d) all of the above

ANSWERS

1. d
2. b
3. d
4. d
5. d

REFERENCES

1. Dolan MG. Emergency care: planning for the worst. *Athl Ther Today*.1998;3(1):12-13.
2. Andersen JC, Courson RW, Kleiner DM, McLoda TA. National Athletic Trainers' Association position statement: emergency planning in athletics. *J Athl Train*. 2002;37(1):99-104.
3. Herbert DL. *Legal Aspects of Sports Medicine*. Canton, OH: Professional Reports Corp; 1990:160-167.
4. Herbert DL. Do you need a written emergency response plan? *Sports Med Stand Malpract Rep*. 1999;11:S17-S24.
5. Courson RW, Duncan K. *The Emergency Plan in Athletic Training Emergency Care*. Boston, MA: Jones and Bartlett; 2000.
6. Courson RW, Roberts WO, Mosesso VN Jr, Link MS, Maron BJ. Inter-association task force recommendations on emergency preparedness and management of sudden cardiac arrest in high school and college athletic programs: a consensus statement. *J Athl Train*. 2007; 42(1):143-158.
7. Potter B, Martin RD. Testing the emergency action plan in athletics. *Athl Ther Today*. 2009;14(6):29-32.
8. Kleinknecht v Gettysburg College, 989 F2d 1360 (3rd Cir 1993).
9. Kleiner DM. Emergency management of athletic trauma: roles and responsibilities. *Emerg Med Serv*. 1998;10:33-36.
10. Arneim DD, Prentice WE. *Principles of Athletic Training*. 9th ed. Madison, WI: WCB/McGraw-Hill Inc; 1997.
11. National Safety Council. *First Aid and CPR*. 4th ed. Sudbury, MA: Jones and Bartlett; 2001.
12. Rubin A. Emergency equipment: what to keep on the sidelines. *Phys Sportsmed*. 1993;21(9):47-54.
13. American Heart Association. Guidelines 2017 for cardiopulmonary resuscitation and emergency cardiovascular care: international consensus on science. *Curr Emerg Cardiovasc Care*. 2017.
14. Drezner JA, Rao AL, Heistand J, Bloomingdale MK, Harmon KG. Effectiveness of emergency response planning for sudden cardiac arrest in United States high schools with automated external defibrillators. *Circulation*. 2009;120(6):518-525.
15. Marenco JP, Wang PJ, Link MS, Homoud MK, Estes MNA 3rd. Improving survival from sudden cardiac arrest: the role of the automated external defibrillator. *JAMA*. 2000;285:1193-1200.
16. National Athletic Trainers' Association. Establishing communication with EMTs. *NATA News*. June 1994:4-9.
17. Feld F. Technology and emergency care. *Athl Ther Today*. 1997;2(5):28.
18. Ray R. *Management Strategies in Athletic Training*. Champaign, IL: Human Kinetics; 2000.
19. Potter, B. Developing professional relationships with emergency medical services providers. *Athl Ther Today*. 2006;11(3):46-47.
20. Casa DJ, Guskiewicz KM, Anderson SA, et al. National Athletic Trainers' Association position statement: preventing sudden death in sports. *J Athl Train*. 2012; 47(1):96-118.
21. Swartz EE, Boden BP, Courson RW, et al. National Athletic Trainers' Association position statement: acute management of the cervical spine-injured athlete. *J Athl Train*. 2009;44(3):306-331.
22. National Athletic Trainers' Association. Official Statement on Athletic Healthcare Provider "Time Outs" Before Athletic Events. http://www.nata.org/official-statements. Accessed January 27, 2015.
23. Robert Morris University. Athletics Emergency Action Plan and Standard Operating Procedures for 2017-18. Athletic Training Handbook. 2017.
24. ATC Spotters. Another Set of Eyes for Injuries. NFL Football Operations. https://operations.nfl.com/the-game/gameday-behind-the-scenes/atc-spotters/. August, 2018. Accessed June 2, 2019.

2

Mass Casualty Incidents

Francis Feld, DNP, CRNA, LAT, ATC, NRP

Chapter Key Words

- Active shooter
- Mass casualty incident
- Triage

Chapter Scenario

It is Friday night, and the high school football game is between 2 long-standing rivals. The game 1 year ago ended on a controversial call, and the home team is seeking to avenge the loss. The student section is exceptionally boisterous, and the stadium is full. As the teams line up for the opening kickoff, a railing in front of the student section gives way, and 20 to 25 students fall approximately 8 feet onto the turf in a tangled mass of humanity.

The ambulance crew on the scene consists of 2 paramedics and 1 emergency medical technician (EMT) in the opposite corner of the field. The crew immediately grabs the equipment and runs toward the incident. The senior medic takes command while the second medic and the EMT start to triage the students for injuries. The commander contacts county dispatch, reports the incident, and requests a second service medic unit plus the on-duty supervisor. Dispatch is also informed that after determining the total number of injuries, a county mass casualty incident (MCI) may be declared. This declaration would bring a third ambulance from the home service, plus 5 additional ambulances from mutual aid companies.

Several off-duty ambulance personnel and nurses come from the stands to assist the crew, and the school principal is also on the scene to gather the names of all the students who fell for risk-management purposes. A total of 22 students fell, and although there were many bumps and bruises, only 2 need transport to a hospital: 1 for an arm fracture, and the other for a laceration requiring sutures. The staff on the scene manages all minor injuries while the second ambulance transports both students to the hospital. Parents are contacted for all students, although many are already there. After all are treated and released to a parent or responsible adult, the members of the crew thank all who helped and return to their position for the game. The referee had stopped the kickoff when he observed the incident and had sent both teams to the sidelines until the issue was resolved. The total delay was approximately 20 minutes, and neither coach complained.

Scenario Resolution

The school emergency action plan (EAP) for this venue did not anticipate the possibility of a railing collapse, but the response was well-managed because of the strength of the local emergency medical services (EMS) agency. Had additional off-duty personnel and nurses not responded from the stands, the athletic trainers from both teams would have been pressed into service and assisted the on-site EMS crew. The game had been delayed, and athletic trainers can handle the soft tissue injuries seen in this incident. Also, the referee had stopped the game and sent the teams to the

Feld F., Gorse KM, Blanc RO
Non-Orthopedic Emergency Care in Athletics (pp 9-13).

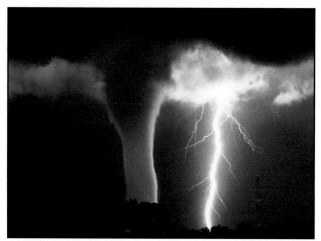

Figure 2-1. Natural disasters.

sidelines. The incident commander had not recognized this until the referee contacted him and indicated that EMS personnel were to take their time and handle the incident thoroughly. The game would not start until the event was resolved, and the referee did not care how long that took. The EAP was updated afterwards to allow for an MCI.

INTRODUCTION

Chapter 1 of this book examined the EAP and how it is developed specific to the venue and in conjunction with local EMS personnel. The chapter takes a strategic approach and considers how to prepare for handling serious injuries and events that will require external resources. Chapter 2 examines the issue from a tactical approach and deals with handling events with multiple patients who will require multiple external resources for mitigation.

An MCI is any event that produces more patients than local EMS can handle. In some resource-strapped communities, this could be a motor vehicle crash with 2 patients, whereas in large urban areas, EMS can handle 50 patients without calling for mutual aid assistance. Although MCIs can be either natural or man-made, the following basic tenets of MCI management apply:

- determine the nature of the incident and its impact on injury profile,
- ascertain the number of injured,
- triage,
- provide initial treatment,
- notify hospitals of the event,
- package and transport the injured,
- clean up, and
- debrief.

Natural MCIs (Figure 2-1) include hurricanes, tornadoes, floods, and fires, whereas man-made MCIs deal with

violence from shootings, stabbings, and bombings. Any of these events can impact athletic venues, and the athletic trainer may be the first health care professional on the scene. Starting the triage process and determining the total number of patients will provide invaluable assistance to responding public safety agencies. If the athletic trainer is to fulfill this role, it must be in conjunction with local agencies and described in the EAP. The athletic trainer must be readily identified as a first responder and have the appropriate equipment for initial management of severe bleeding. Damage from natural MCIs is so widespread that schools usually are closed, and athletic events are suspended. This chapter will mostly examine response to man-made MCIs.

Triage

Triage means *to sort* and is a technique used to determine the number and severity of injuries. The art of triage has been developed by military medicine in battlefield conditions and has significantly reduced battlefield mortalities. Triage is a dynamic process and should be repeated frequently throughout the event, as patient conditions may deteriorate. Many systems are used throughout the country, and the athletic trainer should use the same system used by local EMS. Any triage system divides patients into 4 categories: minor (green), delayed (yellow), immediate (red), and expectant (black).

Minor patients are considered walking wounded and can be transported en masse after all other patients are handled. Delayed patients have injuries that require significant medical treatment, but a slight delay will not cause their condition to worsen. Immediate patients have life- or limb-threatening injuries that require rapid transport. Expectant patients are those with injuries either incompatible with life or so severe that death is imminent and almost certain. Expending limited resources treating these patients may result in delaying treatment and transport of immediate patients and result in the death of many instead of just one. This is a difficult decision and requires unique characteristics in the triage officer.

A commonly used system is the Simple Triage and Rapid Transport (START), which was developed in California by the Newport Beach Fire Department in conjunction with Hoag Hospital (Figure 2-2). Although no system is perfect, START has the advantage of simplicity and concentrates on respiratory status, perfusion, and level of consciousness. Triage tags are attached to each patient, indicating status and providing treatment and transport information to responders. Again, there is no perfect triage tag, and unless EMS either uses or trains with the tags on a continuous basis, their utility is suspect and can lead to confusion and delay.

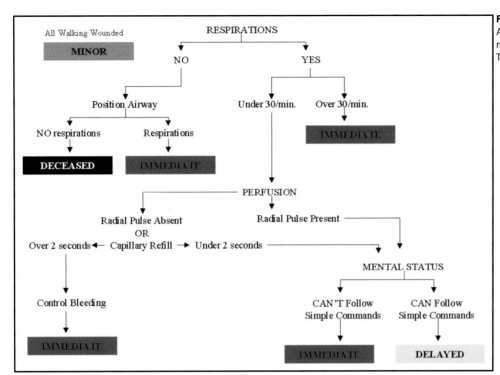

Mass Casualty Incident Management

Following the terrorist attacks of September 11, 2001, the need for a universal command system became apparent, and the federal government developed the National Incident Management System (NIMS).[1] NIMS is used by virtually every public safety agency in the United States. The system can be used not only for large-scale events such as hurricanes, but also for simple events such as a car crash with multiple patients, a house fire, and a railing collapse at a high school stadium. The system can be expanded to meet the needs of the incident, but also simplified for smaller incidents. Although every incident might differ slightly, NIMS uses personnel in the following positions:

- Incident Command (IC). The IC has ultimate authority over all aspects of the response. When multiple agencies are involved (eg, police, fire, EMS), a unified command system may be established with senior leaders of each service, but 1 individual has the final authority. The IC may have deputies and other assistants to complete delegated tasks.
- Operations (OPS). The operations officer manages incident mitigation. OPS can designate officers to handle triage, treatment, transportation, and staging. OPS reports directly to the IC.
- Planning. The planning section predicts needs and communicates the needs to the IC.
- Logistics. Logistics obtains and delivers supplies and equipment to the areas of need.

- Administration and Finance. This section keeps track of costs incurred, including supplies and personnel, as well as any other human resource matters.

Although only very large incidents require every component of NIMS, components are seen in every MCI incident, and the EAP must consider how school personnel will mesh with the local response to an incident. In the case of schools, the senior school official would work with the IC, whereas a school athletic trainer might be detailed to the OPS officer. NIMS is fluid, and although the skeletal frame is consistent across all incidents, the body of the system matches the response. Small incidents do not require filling every position, and 1 person can handle multiple tasks.

NIMS training consists of 4 online courses available through the Federal Emergency Management Agency, plus 2 classroom courses designed for supervisory personnel. The online courses are free of charge and can be completed in a few hours.

Incidents Involving Violence

It is unfortunate that mass shootings in schools and other public places have become commonplace in the United States. It is pointless to report the numbers of shootings, because they increase almost daily, and any epidemiologic values are outdated as soon as they are published. Every school in the country has a plan for an active shooter response, and athletic personnel must familiarize themselves with the plan and how they are to respond, especially if they are not full-time employees. Athletic trainers working in venues other than schools, such as clinics, should determine whether the venue has a plan and, if not, work with administration to develop and practice a plan.

Several commonly used active shooter response plans are available, and all have their merits. Any plan used must consider local resources and capabilities. All plans use the same basic tenets, although nomenclature may differ.

1. RUN. Leave the building as soon as an event is recognized and take as many people with you as possible. Leave belongings behind, and if somebody freezes and will not move, leave him or her. Have a designated rally point outside the building where all can assemble safely and start identifying those who escaped.

2. HIDE. If the shooter is nearby, shelter in place. Lock and barricade the door. Turn off all cell phones, lights, and radios, and maintain strict silence. The shooter is attracted to sound and is looking for targets. Open the door only when you are certain police are on the other side. Make no sudden movement when initially interacting with police.

3. FIGHT. As a last resort, attack the shooter. Loudly scream, and throw any large objects available, such as books or balls, at the shooter for distraction. The shooter is looking for easy targets and may retreat if confronted by large numbers of people rushing and throwing things at him or her.

It is important to understand how police will respond to the incident. This response may vary by locality, but the basic components are the same. Prior to 1999, the standard police response was for the first officers on the scene to establish a perimeter and prevent the shooter from escaping. Entry into the building and capture of the shooter was the function of a Special Weapons and Tactics (SWAT) team. The shootings at Columbine High School in Colorado changed this response.[2] Only very large police departments can afford a full-time SWAT team, and most departments rely on specially trained officers who may be off-duty when responding. This ultimately results in a significant delay while the shooting continues. Most police departments have armed patrol officers with assault rifles instead of shotguns, and those officers are now capable and trained to make entry before the arrival of SWAT, which has been renamed Special Response Team.

Although many departments require a team of 4 patrol officers to make entry, many departments are adopting a 1- or 2-person entry team out of necessity. The object of the entry team is to find and eliminate the shooter. The entry team will not treat the wounded or help anyone escape. Every person the team encounters is considered a suspect, so always have your empty hands up in the air and make no sudden movements. Follow the team's instructions to the letter, and quickly provide any first-hand information you may have about the shooter. When past the entry team, exit the building quickly—again, with your empty hands in the air. Police will search all who evacuate and then direct them to a secure area for debriefing.

The response of EMS to these incidents has also evolved. Traditionally, EMS waited in a safe area and entered the building only after police declared the scene safe. Many EMS agencies have obtained special tactical medicine training for paramedics and will now enter the building before the threat is eliminated. These medics may be armed, and their first priority is assisting any police officer who may be wounded. They will start initial triage and treatment of victims as soon as possible and coordinate the response of additional EMS personnel.

The American College of Surgeons recognized the need to improve survivability following mass shootings, and, in conjunction with multiple law enforcement, EMS, and medical organizations, held a series of meetings in Hartford, Connecticut, to address the issue. The results are a series of published papers that deal with medical care during and after a violent MCI. These papers are known as the Hartford Consensus and are a must read for anyone who is developing a mass violence response plan.[3-7] The Stop the Bleed campaign, which teaches health care providers and lay persons how to manage life-threatening hemorrhage, arose from the Hartford Consensus, and all citizens should avail themselves of the training. The "See Something, Say Something" adage that arose from terrorist attacks has evolved into "See Something, Say Something, DO Something." The hemorrhage control as taught in the Stop the Bleed campaign is covered in a subsequent chapter of this text.

Chapter Summary

Athletic trainers must ensure that the EAP in place for their institution takes an all-hazard approach and covers all foreseeable events. Geography often plays a part in planning, as a hurricane is likely for Florida and the Gulf Coast but unlikely for Montana. Still, thinking outside the box and planning for an event that would be rare is reasonable. Poor response to an MCI is often directly related to poor planning. Practice and evaluate the EAP at least once per year, and plan for the unexpected.

Chapter Review Questions

1. Define MCI and describe its characteristics.
2. List and define the 4 triage classifications.
3. List 3 components of a standard response to an active shooter situation.
4. What is NIMS?
5. When evacuating a building during an active shooter incident, what should you do?

ANSWERS

1. MCI stands for mass casualty incident and is any event that produces a sufficient number of patients that would overwhelm local resources and require response from mutual aid agencies.

2. Green is for walking wounded, yellow is for those with injuries that will not worsen with delayed transport, red is for those sustaining life- and or limb-threatening injuries that require immediate transport, and black is for those who are already dead or those who will likely die no matter what treatment they receive.

3. Run, hide, and fight.

4. NIMS stands for the National Incident Management System and is a universal command structure for response to MCIs, disasters, and everyday public safety events.

5. Keep your empty hands up in the air, make no sudden movements, and follow police commands precisely.

REFERENCES

1. US Department of Homeland Security. National Incident Management System. March 1, 2004. vet.utk.edu. Accessed September 11, 2018. www.fema.gov/national-incident-management-system.

2. Jacobs LM, Wade D, McSwain NF, et al. Hartford Consensus: a call to action for THREAT, a medical disaster preparedness concept. *J Am Coll Surg.* 2014;218(3):467-475.

3. Jacobs LM, McSwain N, Rotondo M, et al. Joint Committee to create a national policy to enhance survivability from mass casualty shooting events. Improving survival from active shooter events: the Hartford consensus. *Bull Am Coll Surg.* 2013;98(6):14-16.

4. Jacobs LM, McSwain NE, Rotondo MF, et al. Improving survival from active shooter events: The Hartford Consensus. *J Trauma Acute Care Surg.* 2013;74(6):1399-1400.

5. Jacobs LM. Joint committee to create a national policy to enhance survivability from mass casualty shooting events: The Hartford Consensus II. *J Am Coll Surg.* 2014;218(3):476-478.

6. Pons PT, Jerome J, McMullen J. The Hartford Consensus on active shooters: implementing the continuum of prehospital trauma response. *J Emer Med.* 2015;49(6):875-885.

7. Jacobs, LM, Burns, KJ, Langer, G, et. al. The Hartford Consensus: a national survey of the public regarding bleeding control. *J Am Coll Surg.* 2016;222(5):948-955.

3

Substance Abuse

Joseph Andrie, MD; John Panos, MEd, LAT, ATC, EMT; and Matthew Schaffer, MD

CHAPTER KEY WORDS

- Alcohol abuse
- Narcan (naloxone)
- Opioid epidemic
- Stimulant abuse

CHAPTER SCENARIO

At approximately 4:45 pm, the athletic trainer is notified of a stranger wandering in the high school parking lot and a woman who seems to be asleep in a car.

After school hours, the athletic trainer is the go-to person. No security is available. This is every athletic trainer's nightmare, and, assuming the worst, 911 is called to report the situation and activate emergency medical services (EMS). The district's go-bag and automated external defibrillator are brought onto the scene.

When on the scene, 911 is notified of a 30-something male wandering in the parking lot and acting strangely. Upon further investigation, an adult female who is unresponsive to verbal or painful stimulation and who exhibits shallow breathing, pinpoint pupils, and weak radial and carotid pulse is found in a nearby car. Suspecting an overdose, 2 doses of Narcan (naloxone) are given with an Evzio (Kaléo Inc) auto-injector.

Within a short time, police arrive with paramedics who administer additional Narcan intranasally. EMS secures the patient to a stretcher and moves her to the ambulance. Once in the unit, the patient is placed on a cardiac monitor, blood pressure cuff, and pulse oximeter. While vital signs are being assessed, intravenous access is established, and blood glucose levels are obtained. The patient becomes responsive to stimuli, is awake, alert, and oriented and is transported to the local emergency department.

SCENARIO RESOLUTION

Fox Chapel Area School District (Pennsylvania) and state Department of Health protocol/steps were initiated.

1. Call EMS.
2. Check for signs of opioid overdose.
3. Commence rescue breathing/cardiopulmonary resuscitation.
4. Administer Evzio (naloxone) through HCl injection.
5. Continue rescue breathing/cardiopulmonary resuscitation if needed.
6. Administer second dose of naloxone (by EMS upon arrival).
7. Place person in recovery position.
8. Transport to the local medical facility.

Athletic trainers must realize that no matter what time or place, coaches and athletes will call for the athletic trainer for all issues that may arise on campus. This is why all athletic trainers need to be Narcan-trained, and they need to incorporate this training into their school district's

Feld F., Gorse KM, Blanc RO
Non-Orthopedic Emergency Care in Athletics (pp 15-19).

alert, lockdown, inform, counter, evacuate; cardiopulmonary resuscitation; child abuse; sudden cardiac arrest; and concussion recognition preparation.

INTRODUCTION

Substance abuse, particularly opioid and stimulant use, continues to capture national attention for its catastrophic and often deadly effects on adolescents and young adults. Athletes at every age and competition level have been found to use drugs or other substances, whether for performance enhancement or because of underlying substance use disorders. Health professionals who have frequent contact with this population should possess a foundational understanding of the use, misuse, and adverse effects of substance use in athletes. This chapter will focus primarily on opioids, prescription stimulants, and alcohol, as these are the most commonly encountered substances of abuse in clinical practice.

The current opioid epidemic is among the deadliest drug epidemics in American history, representing 66.4% of drug overdoses in the United States in 2016,[1] causing fatalities among individuals younger than 50 years old at a faster pace than the HIV epidemic did at its peak.[2] According to the National Survey on Drug Use and Health,[3] 2.1 million people initiated prescription pain reliever misuse in 2016. Even more astonishingly, 19.8% of this population were between the ages of 12 and 17, and 27.4% were between the ages of 18 and 25. This epidemic is fueled largely by the prevalence of prescription opioids.[4] Young athletes are especially prone to substance abuse, with their first exposure to opioids often coming through prescriptions received for sports-related injuries.[5] Through misuse of opioid pain medications, athletes may mask the pain of injury, allowing them to resume playing before the injury is fully healed.

Stimulant medications also have recently seen an increase in misuse. Reported in the 2016 National Survey on Drug Use and Health, 1.4 million people initiated prescription stimulant misuse, with 44.9% of this population being between the ages of 18 and 25, and another 17.7% between the ages of 12 and 17. Most commonly, stimulant medications (eg, amphetamines) are prescribed for treatment of attention-deficit/hyperactivity disorder (ADHD), the most common neuropsychiatric disorder of childhood.[6] Studies have demonstrated a relationship between Adderall (amphetamine and dextroamphetamine mixed salts) use and participation in organized sports, particularly high-contact sports.[7] Aside from their neuropsychiatric action, stimulants can cause adverse cardiovascular effects when combined with physiologic stresses and sports. Those providing care to athletes of all levels must be aware of the potential for cardiovascular emergencies caused by concurrent use or misuse of stimulant medications and physical exertion.[8]

Despite recent surges in opioid and stimulant use among the general and athletic populations, alcohol remains the most commonly used psychoactive drug[9] and is the most widely used drug among the athletic population. In fact, up to 88% of intercollegiate American athletes have been reported to use alcohol.[10] Interestingly, several studies have demonstrated that sport participation is positively associated with greater alcohol use during adolescence and into early adulthood.[11] With this in mind, it is imperative to equip health care professionals who care for athletes with the knowledge base to identify, evaluate, and respond to emergencies caused by the consumption of alcohol before, during, and after athletic events.

Opioids

Misuse and Use in Athletics

In 2017, the opioid crisis in America reached the level of a public health emergency, highlighting the devastation it has caused throughout the country. Athletes are not immune to this crisis, and, in fact, some athletes may fall into a category that places them at higher risk of opioid misuse and abuse.[12] Young athletes in high-contact sports, such as wrestling, football, and ice hockey, are at greater risk to engage in nonmedical use of prescription opioids.[1] The driving factor is thought to be due to the greater risk of injury and subsequent requirement for pain medications, often involving opioid prescriptions. This increased risk of early exposure to opioid pain medications, combined with the stress associated with high-level competition, places athletes into a particularly vulnerable position for development of opioid misuse and abuse.

Pharmacology and Physiology

The term *opioid* refers to a large group of drugs, including naturally derived alkaloids from poppy seeds such as morphine and codeine, as well as their semisynthetic derivatives (eg, fentanyl) and synthetic derivatives (eg, methadone). Opioids act on 3 major classes of receptors that are widely distributed throughout the central and peripheral nervous system, as well as many other organ systems, including the gastrointestinal tract. When opioids interact with tissues in the human body, they reduce the release of neurotransmitters and primarily cause inhibition of physiologic processes, most notably decreasing transmission of pain. Routes of administration include oral, sublingual, intravenous, intranasal, transdermal, and rectal.

Recognition on the Sidelines

Opioids can have physiologic effects on the human body that manifest as both obvious and subtle physical examination findings. Neurologically, opioid use can result in changes in mood and affect, called *dysphoria*. At higher doses, especially in somewhat opioid-naïve patients, sedation can be achieved. Athletes may become less aware or less responsive than normal. At extremes of use, patients can become sedated. On examination, patients under the influence of opioids will develop pinpoint pupils, called *miosis*. Seizures have also been known to occur at lower thresholds in people who are actively using opioids.

Related to neurologic effects, opioid use can cause respiratory depression. This refers to the decreased respiratory rate and drive that occur in those under the influence of opioids. This can lead to poor ventilation and retention of carbon dioxide, leading to a respiratory acidosis, which can have deleterious effects during physical performance.

Opioids also cause changes in the gastrointestinal system, including nausea, vomiting, and constipation. This is due to overall slowing of gastrointestinal motility.

Finally, opioids can have cardiovascular effects. In line with depression of the pulmonary, gastrointestinal, and neurologic systems, opioids can also cause depression of the cardiovascular system. This manifests as decreased heart rate, called *bradycardia*.

Naloxone

Naloxone (Narcan, Evzio) is a medication used to block the effects of opioids and is therefore given in emergency settings when opioid overdose is suspected. It is a nonselective and competitive opioid receptor antagonist, rapidly displacing opioid medications from their receptors and reversing their effects. To highlight its ability to save lives, naloxone has been placed on the World Health Organization's List of Essential Medicines. Naloxone can be given intravenously, intramuscularly, or intranasally. When given intravenously or intranasally, effects are typically seen after 2 minutes. The intramuscular route has a time-to-peak effect of 5 minutes. When administered, the effects last between 30 minutes and 1 hour. Sequential dosing may be considered every 2 to 3 minutes if the desired effect is not achieved after initial administration.

Stimulants

Prevalence Among Athletes

The category of stimulants is broad and can include prescriptions amphetamines, such as those used for ADHD, and recreational stimulants. Recreational stimulants can be both legal, such as caffeine, or illegal, such as methamphetamines or Ecstasy (3,4-methylenedioxy-methamphetamine, or MDMA). The National Collegiate Athletic Association has acknowledged that the number of student-athletes testing positive for stimulant medications has increased 3-fold in recent years.[13] In addition, a 2008 study found that 8% of Major League Baseball players in 2009 obtained exemptions for stimulants.[14] The diagnosis of ADHD in children and adolescents has increased in recent years, leading an increase in stimulants use among young athletes. Sports medicine physicians and athletic trainers should identify athletes who are prescribed stimulants and monitor them for adverse effects.[15]

Pharmacology and Physiology

In general, a stimulant is a psychoactive substance with central nervous system stimulation and mood-altering properties. Exact mechanisms of action are complicated, but most likely involve inhibition of neurotransmitter uptake, specifically monoamine, at the nerve–nerve junction. Stimulants can be consumed orally, intranasally, intravenously, or through inhalation.

Recognition on the Sidelines

As the name implies, stimulants tend to speed up most body processes.

In the cardiovascular system, stimulants cause increased heart rate, thereby increasing cardiovascular output. Increased cardiovascular output, combined with increased systemic vascular resistance, causes increases in blood pressure. Stimulant use can also lead to palpitations, heart attack, and fatal cardiac arrhythmias. Any athlete known to use stimulants who suddenly collapses on the sidelines should be attached to an automated external defibrillator immediately, as the chance of fatal arrhythmia causing the collapse is high.

In addition to cardiovascular signs and symptoms, stimulants also contribute to neurologic changes, including confusion, increased alertness, psychoses, and, at the extreme, seizures. Athletes combining stimulants with rigorous physical activity, such as sporting events, are also at increased risk of developing rhabdomyolysis, which is rapid breakdown of skeletal muscle, leading to renal failure, lactic acidosis, and dehydration. Athletes using stimulants may also be noted to have excessive sweating.

Alcohol

Prevalence Among Athletes

Alcohol is the most widely used drug among the athletic population, including almost 90% of collegiate athletes.[10] *Alcohol use disorder*, as defined by the Diagnostic and Statistical Manual of Mental Disorders-5, is separated into mild, moderate, and severe subclassifications. The diagnosis of alcohol use disorder is beyond the scope of this text, but health care providers should be aware of a wide spectrum of alcohol use in adolescents and adults. In particular, young men between the ages of 18 and 24 are at an increased risk of problem drinking.[10] This is also notably the age group in which sport participation is the highest.

Pharmacology and Physiology

Alcohol, or ethanol, is a naturally occurring substance created by the fermentation of sugars by yeasts. It is legally available in many forms, including beer, wine, and liquor. Alcohol is a psychoactive substance and functions as a central nervous system depressant.

Recognition on the Sidelines

Alcohol is considered an performance-impairing, or ergolytic, drug. As such, alcohol intoxication in athletes can predispose them to deleterious physiologic effects and possibly leads to the need for emergency care on the sideline.

Alcohol concentrations over 100mg/dL weaken the pumping force of the heart, even in young, otherwise healthy individuals, predisposing athletes to cardiovascular insufficiency. This may manifest as lessened exercise tolerance and greater likelihood of syncopal events.[10] Alcohol can affect the electrical system of the heart as well by causing myocardial irritability, resulting in potentially fatal atrial arrhythmias.[10]

In athletes who have a history of exercise-induced asthma, use of alcohol has been identified as a precipitating factor for acute exacerbations.[10]

It is well-known and understood that alcohol use impairs judgment and slows reaction time. Therefore, alcohol use during sporting events that require complex coordination and judgment can increase risk of injury.

Alcohol has been reported as a significant factor in spinal injuries occurring in recreational sports by inhibiting depth perception. Balance also is greatly diminished when the vestibular system is impaired by alcohol, further increasing risk of injury.

Response to Suspected Substance Abuse or Intoxication

Regardless of the suspected substance, it is crucial for athletic organizations at all levels to have a policy in place directing first-line caregivers with the proper actions to take in emergency situations involving substance use.[12] In the event of hemodynamic instability as a result of substance use, the proper basic life support or advanced life support protocol must be followed, including naloxone administration if opioid use is suspected.

Appropriately addressing sideline emergencies relating to substance use and misuse begins with prevention. Several state interscholastic athletic associations have published recommendations for monitoring substance use in athletes. Most of these policies have centered on the opioid crisis but could easily be adapted to other substances. A proactive approach to prevention of substance misuse must involve all members of the sports medicine team. This includes student–athletes, parents or guardians, coaches, athletic trainers, and sports medicine physicians.

A proactive approach to substance misuse includes the following key facets:

- Providing education and awareness at the organizational level to athletes, parents/guardians, and coaches.
- Supporting educational efforts within the school community.
- Employing lower risk, first-line analgesic treatment strategies, such as nonsteroidal anti-inflammatory drugs, acetaminophen, local anesthetics, and cryotherapy, and reserving opioids for more serious injuries or extreme pain.
- Avoiding direct prescribing or dispensing of opioid prescriptions to athletes and avoiding opioid administration in unsupervised environments.
- In school environments, ensuring that prescribers or parents/guardians notify the school nurse or athletic trainer regarding persons who are prescribed stimulants or opioids; school policies should facilitate this process.
- Developing a directed policy for the athletic organization that can be implemented on the sideline regarding athletes suspected to be under the influence of a substance before, during, or after sport participation.
- Making long-term referral resources readily available to athletes to treat not only the acute phase of intoxication, but also the possibility of underlying addiction. This includes a patient-centered approach to treatment.

CHAPTER SUMMARY

Substance use and abuse in athletics are becoming increasingly prevalent, and it is vital that health professionals who care for athletes at every level have a foundational understanding of these substances' effects on performance, as well as their adverse effects. Opioids, both prescription and non-prescription, are the fastest growing drug of abuse and are widely prevalent among athletes. Athletes are at higher risk for traumatic injury, making it more likely that they will receive prescription opioid pain medications. Naloxone is a life-saving reversal agent for opioid overdose and should be administered rapidly in the field.

In addition to opioids, alcohol continues to be the most used drug globally. It is an ergolytic agent, meaning that it has negative effects on performance and can predispose athletes to musculoskeletal injury as well as cardiac and pulmonary adverse effects. Stimulants, mainly prescription agents for the treatment of ADHD, are also prevalent among adolescent athletes. Although primarily neuropsychiatric in their effects, stimulants can cause adverse cardiovascular and heat tolerance effects when combined with physiologic stress, such as sports participation. Regardless of the substance involved, athletic organizations at every level must have a protocol in place to identify athletes who are using substances, whether prescribed or recreationally.

CHAPTER REVIEW QUESTIONS

1. While covering a high school football game, one of the athletes is noted to be less alert than usual, more agitated, and complaining of being nauseated. When examining him, the athletic trainer notes his pupils are smaller than normal. Which substance is this athlete most likely under the influence of?
   a) amphetamine
   b) alcohol
   c) opioid
   d) nicotine

2. Which of the following questions is true regarding naloxone?
   a) it is used primarily as a reversal agent when stimulant overdose is suspected
   b) it can be given intravenously only
   c) it can be given every 2 to 3 minutes if no effect is seen after initial administration
   d) it typically takes 30 minutes to see a true effect

3. Key facets to addressing substance use at the organizational level include which of the following?
   a) providing education and awareness at the organizational level to guardians/parents
   b) attempting to use conservative measures for treatment of pain, including nonsteroidal anti-inflammatory drugs, acetaminophen, local agents, and cryotherapy
   c) avoiding administering opioid medications to adolescents in an uncontrolled environment
   d) all the above

ANSWERS

1. c
2. c
3. d

REFERENCES

1. Veliz PT, Boyd C, Mccabe SE. Playing Through Pain: Sports Participation and Nonmedical Use of Opioid Medications Among Adolescents. *American Journal of Public Health.* 2013;103(5). doi:10.2105/ajph.2013.301242.
2. Salam M. The Opioid Epidemic: A Crisis Years in the Making. *The New York Times.* October 26, 2017.
3. National Survey on Drug Use and Health (NSDUH). National Survey on Drug Use and Health. https://nsduhweb.rti.org/resp-web/homepage.cfm. Accessed October 17, 2018.
4. Spencer K. Opioids on the Quad. *The New York Times.* October 30, 2017.
5. Welsh JW, Tretyak V, Rappaport N. The Opioid Crisis and Schools-A Commentary. *Journal of School Health.* 2018;88(5):337-340. doi:10.1111/josh.12617.
6. White RD, Harris GD, Gibson ME. Attention Deficit Hyperactivity Disorder and Athletes. *Sports Health.* 2013;6(2):149-156. doi:10.1177/1941738113484697.
7. Veliz P, Boyd CJ, Mccabe SE. Nonmedical Use of Prescription Opioids and Heroin Use Among Adolescents Involved in Competitive Sports. *Journal of Adolescent Health.* 2017;60(3):346-349. doi:10.1016/j.jadohealth.2016.09.021.
8. Veliz P, Boyd C, Mccabe SE. Adolescent Athletic Participation and Nonmedical Adderall Use: An Exploratory Analysis of a Performance-Enhancing Drug. *Journal of Studies on Alcohol and Drugs.* 2013;74(5):714-719. doi:10.15288/jsad.2013.74.714.
9. Barnes MJ. Alcohol: Impact on Sports Performance and Recovery in Male Athletes. *Sports Medicine.* 2014;44(7):909-919. doi:10.1007/s40279-014-0192-8.
10. O'Brien CP, Lyons F. Alcohol and the Athlete. *Sports Med.* 2000;29(5):295-300.
11. Kwan M, Bobko S, Faulkner G, Donnelly P, Cairney J. Sport participation and alcohol and illicit drug use in adolescents and young adults: A systematic review of longitudinal studies. *Addictive Behaviors.* 2014;39(3):497-506. doi:10.1016/j.addbeh.2013.11.006.
12. NJSIAA Issues Recommendations to Combat Opioid Use Among Athletes. *NJSIAA.* 2016.
13. Buckman JF, Farris SG, Yusko DA. A national study of substance use behaviors among NCAA male athletes who use banned performance enhancing substances. *Drug and Alcohol Dependence.* 2013;131(1-2):50-55. doi:10.1016/j.drugalcdep.2013.04.023.
14. Reardon, C, Creado, S. Drug abuse in athletes. *Substance Abuse and Rehabilitation.* 2014;95. doi: 10.2147/sar.s53784.
15. Wolfe ES, Madden KJ. Evidence-Based Considerations and Recommendations for Athletic Trainers Caring for Patients With Attention-Deficit/Hyperactivity Disorder. *Journal of Athletic Training.* 2016;51(10):813-820. doi:10.4085/1062-6050-51.12.11.

4

Cardiovascular Emergencies

Jason Ferderber, MD and Vincent Mosesso Jr, MD

CHAPTER KEY WORDS

- Commotio cordis
- Hypertrophic cardiomyopathy
- Supraventricular tachycardia
- Wolff-Parkinson-White syndrome

CHAPTER SCENARIO

A 20-year-old male college basketball player collapses during a game while running down the court. He then appears to have seizure-like activity, with occasional gasping for air. He had a preparticipation physical before the season, with no concerning findings, and he has no family history of sudden cardiac death or arrhythmias.

The basketball player was assumed to be in cardiac arrest due to the sudden collapse and irregular breathing; thus, the athletic trainer started cardiopulmonary resuscitation (CPR) immediately. Another staff member at the school retrieved the automated external defibrillator (AED), and, after placement of the pads, a shock was recommended. The athletic trainer administered the shock and immediately resumed CPR. In 2 minutes, a pulse check revealed a bounding femoral pulse. The player soon began breathing on his own.

SCENARIO RESOLUTION

Upon emergency medical services (EMS) arrival, an electrocardiogram (EKG) was obtained that showed prominent Q waves in multiple leads and criteria for left ventricular hypertrophy. Given the clinical situation and EKG findings, hypertrophic cardiomyopathy was suspected. The player was transferred to the hospital, and, after further evaluation by the cardiology team, he had successful placement of an implantable cardioverter defibrillator (ICD) with no further episodes of syncope or cardiac arrest.

INTRODUCTION

This chapter will discuss cardiovascular emergencies that are common or important causes of death and disability in athletes. The focus is on sudden cardiac arrest (SCA), including both congenital and acquired causes, the importance of immediate recognition, and the principles of management. The impact of exercise on short- and long-term cardiovascular health is discussed. Finally, the chapter reviews the most common cardiac dysrhythmias that cause symptoms or sudden death in athletes.

Feld F., Gorse KM, Blanc RO
Non-Orthopedic Emergency Care in Athletics (pp 21-34).
© 2020 Taylor & Francis Group.

TABLE 4-1. FIVE COMMON ELECTROCARDIOGRAM CHANGES SEEN IN ATHLETES

Sinus bradycardia

First-degree atrioventricular block

Incomplete right bundle branch block

Early repolarization changes

Voltage criteria for left ventricular hypertrophy

Cardiac Arrest

Sudden cardiac death (SCD) has become a commonly recognized phenomenon in athletics today. It is defined as death of primary cardiac etiology, occurring within 1 hour of witnessed symptom onset and within 24 hours if the incident is unwitnessed. EKG is the best current screening tool[1]; however, no screening interventions have proven to totally eliminate SCA in athletes.[2] Most individuals have no signs or symptoms prior to the incident, and this is a key reason why prevention and screening are difficult in this population.[3]

An Athlete's Heart

Athletic conditioning is known to cause cardiac remodeling, with corresponding EKG changes, and must be differentiated from pathologic entities.[4] The Seattle criteria were created to assist physicians and health care providers in determining concerning versus normal physiologic EKG findings.[5] Common changes seen on the EKGs of athletes are shown in Table 4-1. Normal exercise results in physiologic left ventricular hypertrophy; however, this should be differentiated from pathologic hypertrophy, such as hypertrophic and hypertensive cardiomyopathy. Eccentric hypertrophy is due to compensation for an increased circulating volume, with creation of sarcomeres in series, with resultant elongation of myocytes. This often develops after dynamic exercise, much like that in football and soccer, causing an increase in the left ventricular cavity. Static exercise, such as weight lifting, causes concentric hypertrophy, with an unchanged size of the left ventricular cavity.[6,7] This is due to new sarcomeres being created in parallel, versus in series, from chronic pressure overload, resulting in a thickened myocardium. Concentric hypertrophy is commonly seen in persons with chronically elevated blood pressure due to the heart having to pump against an increased afterload. The amount of hypertrophy correlates to the risk of fatal arrhythmias and SCD.[7]

Incidence

Most SCAs occur during or immediately after exercise.[3] The incidence of SCA is always a moving target, but ranges between 1 in 65,000 and 1 in 200,000 athlete-years.[8] For high school and college athletes specifically, most recent data have published the death rate to be 1 in 50,000 to 1 in 80,000.[9] Ventricular fibrillation (VF) and pulseless ventricular tachycardia (pVT) are the most common cardiac rhythms identified in out-of-hospital cardiac arrest. Pulseless electrical activity (PEA) is less common with a higher mortality rate.[10]

Etiology

Most sports-related SCDs occur in individuals older than 35 years.[11] In National College Athletic Association athletes, SCA is the leading cause of death during exercise,[12] with the highest rate occurring in male basketball players.[13] Male athletes are more likely to be affected compared to females (male to female ratio 5:1),[14] but survival rates have been relatively similar between the sexes. A recent study found that basketball and football account for more than half of SCAs in the high school and college-aged athlete.[15] In marathon runners, most SCA cases are seen in the final 4 miles of the race.[16] SCA has also been found to occur almost 4 times more commonly in nonorganized athletic activities compared to organized activities, and more than one-third of those cases were due to coronary artery disease (CAD) in individuals 35 to 45 years of age.[17]

The primary causes of SCD are different in athletes who are less than 35 years of age compared to those who older than 35 years of age. In the younger population, a structurally normal heart is the most common finding on autopsy.[3,9,13,18,19] Commonly identified etiologies are shown in Table 4-2.[18-20]

The leading cause of death in athletes is due to SCA and is usually prompted by the increased physiologic demands of exercise in those with preexisting cardiac conditions.[9] More than 80% of the cardiac deaths in athletes have been associated with physical exertion.[21] Multiple case reports have linked anabolic steroid use to cardiac arrest in body builders.[22-24] When referring to patients older than 35 years, most SCDs are caused by CAD, compared to younger individuals, where arrhythmias and inherited abnormalities are more common.[20,25,26] With a 33% increase in the number of Americans over the age of 65 over the past decade, which is expected to double by 2060,[27] SCA could become a more common entity.

Hypertrophic Cardiomyopathy

One of the congenital etiologies linked to SCD in young athletes is hypertrophic cardiomyopathy (HCM), which causes asymmetric thickening of the ventricular septum in 90% of affected individuals, and less commonly involves hypertrophy of the left ventricular wall. Although this

TABLE 4-2. COMMON ETIOLOGIES FOR SUDDEN CARDIAC DEATH IN INDIVIDUALS YOUNGER THAN 35 YEARS OF AGE [18-20]	
• HCM	• Idiopathic left ventricular hypertrophy
• Coronary artery anomalies	• Dilated cardiomyopathy
• ARVC	• Myocarditis
• Long QT syndrome	• Aortic dissection
• Brugada syndrome	• WPW
Abbreviations: ARVC, arrhythmogenic right ventricular cardiomyopathy; HCM, hypertrophic cardiomyopathy; WPW, Wolff-Parkinson-White	

condition is inherited in an autosomal-dominant pattern, with an average presentation in the third decade of life, it unfortunately can also occur sporadically without any preceding family history.

Unlike other causes of hypertrophy, in which myocytes grow in an orderly and uniform fashion, patients with HCM suffer from a genetic mutation that causes myocyte disarray, with disorderly cell growth and fibrosis. This leads to diastolic dysfunction and arrhythmias. Figure 4-1 shows classic changes that can be seen on EKG in these patients. The first sign or symptom of HCM may be VF, resulting in SCD. A history of exertional syncope or a positive family history of SCD should prompt further cardiac workup. This condition is more challenging to recognize because these patients routinely have a normal physical examination and are asymptomatic.[7,28]

HCM can occur with or without outflow tract obstruction. In patients with no outflow tract obstruction, cardiac hypertrophy causes increased wall stiffness and diastolic dysfunction. The resultant elevated end-diastolic pressure creates back pressure throughout the cardiopulmonary system, leading to dyspnea on exertion. Patients with outflow tract obstruction differ in their pathophysiology. A hypertrophied septum causes obstruction of the lower ventricle outflow tract, which is amplified by high demand and is more so when combined with intravascular volume depletion commonly seen in athletes. This dehydration causes a decrease in the size of the lower ventricle chamber, bringing the hypertrophied septum and anterior leaflet of the mitral valve closer together, resulting in outflow obstruction.[7] This can lead to syncope from transiently decreased cerebral blood flow.

These patients can have exercise-induced cardiac ischemia, which, over time, causes myocardial fibrosis and cell death.[29] This, in combination with the unorganized hypertrophic changes, can predispose an individual to further atrial and ventricular arrhythmias as well as heart failure. The hypertrophy in HCM decreases compliance, which differs from the hypertrophy occurring with a seasoned athlete, who has no focal hypertrophy and maintains a normal left ventricle cavity size, with no left atrial enlargement.[28]

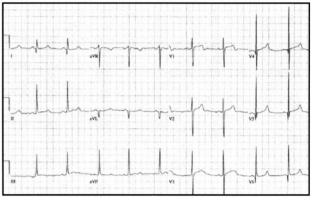

Figure 4-1. Common EKG findings in HCM, including pathologic Q waves and left ventricular hypertrophy.

Beta blockers are the typical therapy for individuals with HCM, improving diastolic filling by decreasing chronotropy and inotropy. They also allow for a decrease in the left ventricular outflow tract pressure gradient.[7,28] However, pharmacologic therapy alone does **not** prevent SCD, which has led to the advent of ICD placement to prevent fatal arrhythmias in these patients.[7,30]

Arrhythmogenic Right Ventricular Cardiomyopathy

Another well-known cause of SCD is arrhythmogenic right ventricular cardiomyopathy (ARVC). ARVC involves the infiltration and replacement of the myocardium and the His-Purkinje bundle with adipose and fibrous tissue, classically in the right ventricle.[29,31] Because of this pathology, it is associated with arrhythmias, heart failure, and SCD.[31] The incidence is highest in the second to fifth decades of life.[32] Patients can have palpitations and syncope; however, unfortunately, SCD can be the first symptom, like many of the other conditions discussed in this chapter.[31] One study found that nearly one-quarter of SCDs that occurred in adolescents and young adults during sports were due to ARVC from an exercise-induced catecholamine increase.[33,34] However, another study found that of the individuals diagnosed with ARVC, most died during

TABLE 4-3. COMMONLY PRESCRIBED QT-PROLONGING MEDICATIONS

• Amiodarone	• Ondansetron
• Fluoroquinolones	• Methadone
• Sulfamethoxazole-Trimethoprim	• SSRIs
• Azithromycin	• TCAs
• Diphenhydramine	• Azole medications

Adapted from Fazio G, Vernuccio F, Grutta G, Re GL. Drugs to be avoided in patients with long QT syndrome: focus on the anaesthesiological management. *World J Cardiol.* 2013;5(4):87-93. doi:10.4330/wjc.v5.i4.87. Abbreviations: SSRIs, selective serotonin reuptake inhibitors; TCAs, tricyclic antipressants

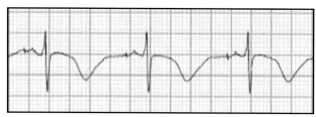

Figure 4-2. Example of a prolonged QT interval.

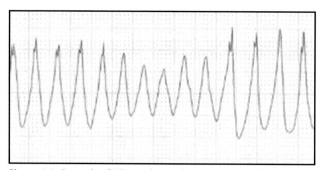

Figure 4-3. Example of TdP, a polymorphic ventricular tachycardia.

normal daily activities or when sedentary.[29] Treatment consists of placement of an ICD.[32,33]

Anomalous Coronary Artery

The presence of an anomalous coronary artery is another cause of SCD in athletes and was found in one study to account for 17% of deaths.[21] The most common abnormality is the occurrence of the left coronary artery origin from the right sinus of Valsalva. This anomalous artery can be constricted when passing between the aorta and pulmonary artery, causing poor cardiac perfusion. The condition can become worse with exertion, given the increased demand on the heart, leading to VF and SCD. Anomalous coronary arteries are ultimately corrected with surgical intervention.[35]

Long and Short QT Syndrome

Long QT syndrome can be congenital or acquired (Figure 4-2). Congenital causes involve loss of function mutations in potassium channels and gain of function mutations in sodium channels.[36] In elite athletes, the prevalence of prolonged QT is 0.4%.[37] Numerous medications, including many antiarrhythmics, antibiotics, and antipsychotics, can cause a prolonged QT interval (Table 4-3).[37] This condition increases the risk of pVT, also known as *Torsades de pointes*, with precipitation into VF.[10] Torsades de pointes is a cardiac rhythm that necessitates prompt treatment (Figure 4-3). The first-line therapy is magnesium sulfate and should be given as soon as possible when this rhythm is identified.

Similar to individuals with a prolonged QT, those with a short QT interval are at risk for arrhythmias, both atrial and ventricular (Figure 4-4). This is caused by a mutation in the potassium channel gene.[35] The first symptom can be atrial fibrillation or, unfortunately, SCD.[38] Patients with this condition are more prone to arrhythmia on exertion due to the catecholamine surge that occurs with the tachycardia of exercise. This causes an even shorter QT interval, leading to deadly arrhythmias.[39]

Brugada Syndrome

Another cardiac ion channelopathy is Brugada syndrome. In this condition, a sodium channel abnormality allows for a greater potassium efflux from cells compared to sodium influx.[40] This causes the well-recognized cove-shaped ST-segment elevation in the right precordial leads on EKG (Figure 4-5). Unfortunately, an athlete's heart can mimic those changes seen in Brugada syndrome; thus, EKG criteria must not be used in isolation for this diagnosis—it must also be based on clinical criteria.[41] Many patients might not even have any EKG changes. However, under the right circumstances, such as a febrile state, hypothermia, hyper- or hypokalemia, hypercalcemia, or cocaine and alcohol toxicity, a patient can experience sudden syncope with decompensation into VF and SCD.[35] Unlike the other

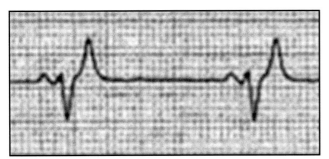

Figure 4-4. Example of a short QT interval.

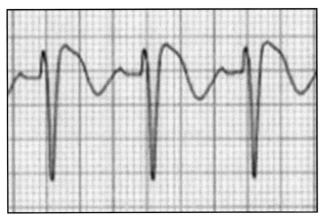

Figure 4-5. EKG showing findings of Brugada syndrome, with cove-shaped ST elevations and T wave changes typically seen in the anterior precordial leads (V1 and V2).

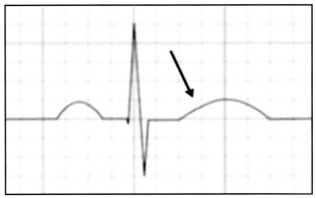

Figure 4-6. Commotio cordis can occur when the chest is impacted over the heart during ventricular repolarization, specifically the upslope of the T wave (arrow).

causes of SCD, this syndrome does not typically present itself during exercise and occurs mostly during rest.[41] Therapy involves placement of an ICD.[35]

Commotio Cordis

Picture a baseball pitcher getting hit in the chest by a line drive. He suddenly collapses and is not moving. What do you do? Commotio cordis occurs with ball-related sports, such as baseball and lacrosse, when there is blunt trauma to the precordium. It has become a more widely recognized etiology of SCD in recent decades. Many of these individuals are found to be in VF and require the same treatment and resuscitation as other patients with this rhythm.[42-44] The location and timing of the impact to the chest is important for development of commotio cordis. The impact must occur on the chest wall directly over the heart during the upslope of the T wave in the cardiac cycle (Figure 4-6).[42,45] Smaller spherical objects are more likely to cause SCA due to a sudden increase in left ventricular pressure, resulting in VF.[45,46] This phenomenon was thought to occur more in younger athletes compared to older individuals due to the increased rate of participation in ball-related sports.[43] However, more recent data suggest that the size of an individual is likely the main factor contributing to the increased incidence in younger athletes.[47] Although previously thought to be shielding, chest protectors have

been shown to not be effective in the prevention of SCA from commotio cordis.[48] Individuals who experience SCA secondary to commotio cordis can resume regular activity if no predisposing cardiac abnormality is identified.[49]

Commotio cordis differs from cardiac contusion, which occurs after blunt trauma, such as a motor vehicle accident, causing structural cardiac damage.[42] This could include contusion of the myocardium, cardiac chamber rupture, or heart valve disruption and can lead to ventricular arrhythmias. Isolated asymptomatic tachycardia also can be associated with myocardial contusion and might be the only sign of cardiac damage.[44] At collision speeds of greater than 50 mph, SCD is more likely to be due to structural cardiac damage rather than commotio cordis.[50]

Myocarditis and Pericarditis

Myocarditis is defined as *inflammation of the heart muscle, ultimately leading to cell death.* The most common etiology is the Coxsackie B virus. Symptoms include chest discomfort, dyspnea, peripheral edema, and fatigue. Cardiogenic shock may occur in severe cases. Treatment is mainly symptomatic with close observation of cardiac function. After clinical resolution, the patient should refrain from vigorous activity for 6 months, have no signs of arrhythmia, and have normal cardiac function prior to return to activity.[51]

Pericarditis involves inflammation of the pericardium that surrounds the heart. Pericarditis is typically idiopathic in origin, but can also be due to a viral infection, much like myocarditis. To make the diagnosis of pericarditis, 2 of 4 clinical criteria are necessary: positional chest pain (eg, pain typically better when sitting than supine), pericardial friction rub, EKG changes (eg, non-vascular distribution of ST elevations and PR segment depressions), and new or worsening pericardial effusion.[52] Both myocarditis and pericarditis can present similarly; thus, a troponin value is useful in determining the diagnosis.

Pericarditis alone should not have any increase in troponin value compared to myocarditis, which should have

TABLE 4-4. NONCARDIAC CAUSES OF SUDDEN DEATH
Asthma
Heat stroke
Acute cerebral disease (cerebral artery rupture, stroke, hyponatremic encephalopathy)
Sickle cell disease
Rhabdomyolysis

a moderately elevated level. However, pericarditis should not be thought of as less dangerous, as these patients can develop cardiac tamponade acutely due to large pericardial effusion and in later stage due to constrictive pericarditis. This is due to poor ventricular filling during diastole from a rigid, fibrous pericardium that can develop after an episode of acute pericarditis and can lead to decreased stroke volume and cardiac output, resulting in hypotension.[7] If pericarditis is diagnosed in an otherwise well-appearing patient, the first-line therapy is non-steroidal anti-inflammatory drugs. Athletes should refrain from physical activity until symptoms have resolved and there are no longer clinical or laboratory signs of disease, such as resolution of pericardial effusion on echocardiogram and normalization of erythrocyte sedimentation rate and C-reactive protein.[53]

Acute Coronary Syndrome

Acute coronary syndrome is more commonly encountered in older athletes due to the higher prevalence of CAD. These patients classically describe a pressure-like sensation on their chest, with pain that radiates to either side of the chest, the jaw, and/or down the left arm. This can be accompanied by nausea, vomiting, diaphoresis, and dyspnea. However, many patient populations—namely women, people with diabetes mellitus, and elderly individuals—can present simply with fatigue and weakness as a first sign of cardiac ischemia. Patients with prior cardiac disease have different signs and symptoms of cardiac ischemia that are often referred to as anginal equivalents, which can be specific to each patient and can vary widely. Medical providers must be highly vigilant in recognizing signs and symptoms of acute coronary syndrome and act swiftly to avoid adverse outcomes.

Noncardiac Causes

Noncardiac causes of SCA include asthma, heat stroke, and cerebral artery rupture (Table 4-4).[8] Although these causes will not be covered in this chapter, they should be considered when thinking of the differential diagnosis in

sudden collapse. As always, the clinical situation should dictate appropriate treatment.

Exercise as a Risk Factor for Sudden Cardiac Death

Regular physical activity has been known to have multiple health benefits, including decreasing the chances of SCD.[11] A dose-response relationship has been observed with physical activity and all-cause mortality. The largest proportional decrease in CV mortality occurs soon after beginning regular physical activity, with even small amounts of exercise significantly decreasing one's cardiovascular risk, as well as aiding in one's memory, attention, and sleep quality. This is important, as individuals can decrease their disease risk within days of starting an exercise regimen.[54]

However, occasional vigorous activity in normally sedentary individuals increases the chance of undergoing an adverse cardiac event.[55,56] One study investigated cardiac dysfunction and associated biomarkers of cardiac injury in marathon runners. Athletes with less training prior to the event were found to have larger increases in their cardiac troponin levels, in addition to increased pulmonary pressures and right ventricular dysfunction on echocardiogram. This right ventricular dysfunction has been reported to occur with endurance exercise, causing structural changes in the heart and possibly leading to fatal arrhythmias.[57]

Management of Cardiac Arrest

Recognition of Sudden Cardiac Arrest

A lot of media attention has been focused on concussions and the subsequent collapse of an athlete after blunt trauma. However, non-contact sudden collapse is a feature of SCA.[58,59] The predisposing arrhythmia causes poor cerebral blood flow and oxygen deprivation to the brain, which can lead to seizures.[8,44] Other observed features that can occur with SCA are a fixed gaze,[58] myoclonic jerks, and agonal or gasping respirations.[8] Syncope related to a vasovagal reflex typically has prodromal symptoms such as nausea, diaphoresis, lightheadedness, and tunnel vision. This is differentiated from ventricular arrhythmia-related syncope, which occurs abruptly without any prodrome. Anyone found unresponsive after sudden collapse without regular breathing should be considered to be in cardiac arrest until proven otherwise.

Emergency Action Plan

Immediate recognition of SCA is critical, and the survival rate depends on the preparedness of those individuals responding at the scene. Emergency action plan (EAP) elements include a communication system, responder training in CPR and AED use, AED access for early defibrillation, availability of emergency equipment, and communication with EMS personnel, as well as the practice and review of actions.[44] All these features must function properly for successful management of an individual in cardiac arrest.

Medical personnel should be familiar with 2 types of defibrillators: AED and manual defibrillator, the latter of which is typically carried by EMS personnel and in hospitals. An AED will self-analyze the heart rhythm and instruct those doing the resuscitation whether to administer a shock. A manual defibrillator requires specific training by health care personnel to analyze the cardiac rhythm and administer appropriate advanced cardiac life support treatment.[60]

More than 90% of SCAs in high school– and college-aged athletes are witnessed. Research has found that when an athletic trainer was on-site at the time of arrest and was involved in the resuscitation, 83% of these athletes survived to hospital discharge. Similar evidence was found that if an on-site AED was available and used during the resuscitation, almost 90% of these athletes survived. Unfortunately, an AED was available on-site in only one-third of cases.[15] A systematic review found that use of an AED by layperson first responders had a greater survival rate than when defibrillation was delayed until arrival by dispatched professional first responders.[62]

A prospective observational study evaluated the effectiveness of high school–based AED programs. More than half the cases were observed in adults (56% versus 44% in students). This study demonstrated a 92% rate of rapid initiation of CPR, with application of a defibrillator occurring in 85% of cases. A shock was delivered in 66% of SCAs, with a 71% survival to hospital discharge.[14] Overall, there has been a trend toward improved survival in recent years for those with SCA,[62] with the hopes of increasing survival with further implementation and practice of school-based AED programs.

Ventricular Fibrillation and Pulseless Ventricular Tachycardia

On many occasions, the recognition and necessary interventions to care for an athlete with SCA are delayed due to apparent signs of life from observers. VF and pVT are common rhythms found in athletes suffering from SCA (Figures 4-7 and 4-8). The first sign could be seizure-like activity involving random myoclonic jerks.[8] It is expected that first responders check for pulses and respirations in a patient with possible cardiac arrest. However, checking for breathing or a pulse has been shown to be inaccurate and time-consuming.[63-65] If there is a lack of a normal breathing pattern, then cardiac arrest should be assumed, and CPR should be started immediately.[8,66-68] The American Heart Association (AHA) stresses that a short time to defibrillation is critical to increasing the chances of survival.[68] A single-person rescuer should activate the EAP and obtain the AED if it can be done easily and in a timely manner prior to beginning CPR. When 2 rescuers are present, one

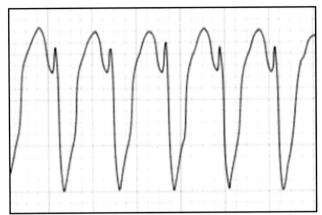

Figure 4-7. Example of monomorphic ventricular tachycardia.

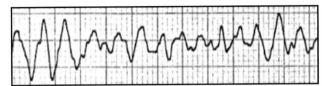

Figure 4-8. Example of ventricular fibrillation.

should begin CPR while the other activates the EAP and retrieves the AED.[66]

The best chance of survival occurs with immediate CPR started within 1 minute, with goal to defibrillation within 2 minutes and no more than 3 to 5 minutes.[44,68,69] Early CPR and defibrillation are imperative to survival, with defibrillation prior to 2 minutes for individuals in pVT or in VF having a 90% return of spontaneous circulation,[8,59] with survival decreasing by 10% for every minute thereafter. Cardiac output during CPR is approximately 10% to 30% of an individual's baseline,[10] reinforcing the urgency of restoring normal cardiac function. When initiating CPR, chest compressions alone are as effective as chest compressions plus ventilation.[70] Halting CPR while giving ventilations has not been shown to be beneficial, with studies showing no difference in 1-month survival between CPR plus ventilations versus CPR alone.[71,72] To assist in increasing CPR rates, in its most recent basic life support guidelines, the AHA recommends compression-only CPR for laypersons and bystanders, as it is easier to perform.[66]

The survival rate to hospital discharge in an out-of-hospital cardiac arrest for various age groups is shown in Table 4-5.[73] The longer the time to defibrillation, the lower the rate of survival.[74] For adults, energy level recommendations vary by manufacturer. We recommend using highest available on the particular model being used. The initial pediatric dose is 2 J/kg, with 4 J/kg in successive shocks. However, if the rescuer is unsure, he or she should use the maximal dose on the specific defibrillator.[10,60] A pulse and rhythm check should occur *prior* to defibrillation and *not* after. After defibrillation, CPR should continue to be administered without a pulse check, as stunning of the

TABLE 4-5. SURVIVAL RATES TO HOSPITAL DISCHARGE IN OUT-OF-HOSPITAL CARDIAC ARREST

AGE GROUP (YEARS)	SURVIVAL RATE (%)
>18	10.6
13-18	23.5
1-12	16.6
<1	6.2

Data from Benjamin EJ, Blaha MJ, Chiuve SE, et al. Heart disease and stroke statistics—2017 update: a report from the American Heart Association. *Circulation*. 2017;135(10):e146-e603.

heart myocardium immediately after defibrillation can occur.

It is necessary for individuals to be properly trained to perform CPR and defibrillation for the survival of those suffering from SCA. A study has shown that school programs teaching these skills improve the survival rate of SCA.[75] The quality of the CPR is imperative as well, with an AHA-recommended chest compression rate of 100 to 120. Of equal importance is the depth and recoil of compressions. A depth of between 2 and 2.5 inches (5 and 6 cm) is recommended, with an equal time ratio of chest compression to chest recoil. Allow full chest wall recoil between compressions.[60] Many sports involve equipment, including shoulder pads, that have been shown to decrease chest compression depth.[76] Therefore, if it would not cause more than a few seconds of delay in initiating CPR, the anterior chest should be exposed, and the chest compressions should be performed directly on the chest. Athletic trainers and other planned responders should be well-versed in rapid removal of equipment.

Pulseless Electrical Activity and Asystole

Defibrillation is indicated for VF and pVT, but what happens when the patient has an organized rhythm but there is still no pulse? This is called *pulseless electrical activity*, or PEA, which can be thought of as having 2 subtypes. True electrical-mechanical dissociation occurs when the intrinsic electrical activity is still functioning properly, but the physical pumping of the heart is not. For example, when an athlete is suffering from hypoxia, the resulting metabolic disturbances hinder the action of the myocardium, but the heart's electrical circuit is preserved. In pseudo-PEA, contractions occur in combination with normal electrical activity, but no pulse is felt.[10]

If the same athlete suffers blunt trauma that causes cardiac tamponade, the heart is still attempting to pump with no intrinsic electrical failure, but no pulse can be felt. In

this theoretical scenario, the chest wall trauma causes cardiac injury and results in blood filling the pericardial space, allowing for buildup of pericardial pressure, resulting in poor diastolic ventricular filling. This causes a decreased stroke volume and cardiac output, leading to systemic hypotension and shock.[7] Ultrasound can be used to differentiate between pathologies.

It is imperative to know the causes of PEA, as certain interventions can be lifesaving prior to EMS arrival or hospital transfer. Think about a football player who gets spear-tackled in the chest. In an instant, he cannot breathe and quickly loses consciousness. You attach the defibrillator, notice that the patient is in PEA, and see chest rise only on the left. Tension pneumothorax is suspected, and needle decompression is done with a large rush of air on insertion, with return of spontaneous circulation. Defibrillation in patients with PEA is not indicated and will not assist in resuscitation. A traditional approach to the evaluation of PEA etiology consists of the "5 Hs and 5 Ts" mnemonic (Table 4-6). In otherwise healthy athletes, many of these issues are unlikely to occur, and, if they do, the best treatment would be to continue basic life support or advanced cardiovascular life support until transfer to the treating facility.

Another rhythm that could be seen is asystole, which exhibits a total lack of cardiac activity with a flat-line appearance on an EKG. Asystole has an extremely poor prognosis and, like PEA, is not amenable to defibrillation. It is **always** the end-product and **not** the cause of cardiac arrest. Many times, it is seen from degradation of VF after myocardial cell death due to an extended duration of hypoxia and acidosis. It can also be from a bradydysrhythmia that occurs from failure of the heart's intrinsic electrical system. Bradycardia itself can be amenable to cardiac pacing if started within minutes.[7] However, no benefit has been found with pacing in asystole, and it is not recommended.[77]

The AHA now revises CPR guidelines on a continuous basis as new research is published. Updated AHA guidelines and recommendations can be found at https://eccguidelines.heart.org/cpr-ecc-guidelines/

Cardiac Arrhythmias, Non-Arrest

Ventricular Tachycardia

Pulseless VT is treated as cardiac arrest. However, if a patient in VT has a pulse, what do you do? VT is the most common form of wide-complex tachycardia (WCT) encountered in clinical practice. It is seen more commonly in individuals with a cardiovascular history, such as a prior myocardial infarction or severe cardiomyopathy. However, electrolyte abnormalities, such as hyperkalemia, cannot be forgotten, as interventions differ greatly. It is often difficult to differentiate VT from supraventricular tachycardia

TABLE 4-6. COMMON CAUSES OF PULSELESS ELECTRICAL ACTIVITY ARREST	
Hs	**Ts**
Hypovolemia	Tension pneumothorax
Hypoxia	Tamponade (cardiac)
Hydrogen ions (acidosis)	Thrombosis (coronary)
Hyper- and hypokalemia	Thrombosis (pulmonary)
Hypothermia	Toxins

(SVT) with aberrancy, the latter of which is the second most common cause of WCT.

When unsure of the diagnosis, **always** assume VT until proven otherwise! With VT, if the patient is clinically unstable, synchronized cardioversion is recommended. Because this is a regular rhythm, it is imperative that the shock be synchronized to avoid putting the heart into VF. If the patient is stable, procainamide or amiodarone has been shown to be effective in converting the heart back to a sinus rhythm. Of course, if an underlying cause, such as hypokalemia, is identified, then that should be corrected as well. Also remember that multifocal VT, or Torsades de pointes, is primarily treated with magnesium intravenously.

Supraventricular Tachycardia

SVT is a fast rhythm that comes from above the ventricles (Figure 4-9). The 2 most commonly encountered etiologies for SVT are atrioventricular nodal reentrant tachycardia (AVNRT) and atrioventricular reentrant tachycardia (AVRT). AVNRT is commonly seen in individuals aged 20 years and older due to a reentry loop involving the atrioventricular (AV) node (Figure 4-10A).

AVRT, on the other hand, is more common in the pediatric population.[78] This occurs through anterograde and/or retrograde electrical impulses through an accessory pathway as well as the AV node (Figure 4-10B). When impulses conduct anterograde (or orthodromic) through the AV node, the ventricular complexes will be narrow with normal morphology. When impulses conduct anterograde through the accessory pathway (and thus antidromic through the AV node), the aberrant ventricular activation results in the classic delta waves and widened QRS complexes seen commonly in Wolff-Parkinson-White (WPW) syndrome.

For SVT of unknown mechanism, the AHA recommends vagal maneuvers, such as Valsalva, carotid massage, and ice to the face. If these are unsuccessful, then adenosine should be administered, which temporarily blocks the AV node to stop conduction to the ventricles, with the hope of halting the reentry loop. When this medication is being considered, one should apply defibrillator pads prior to

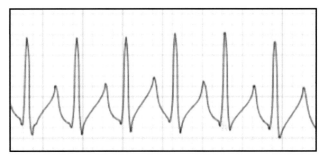

Figure 4-9. Example of supraventricular tachycardia.

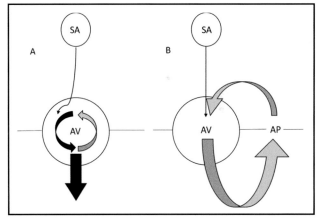

Figure 4-10. AVNRT and AVRT. A. Schematic of AVNRT, with a reentry loop at the AV node (gold arrow). B. Schematic of anterograde AVRT, with an accessory pathway (AP) creating a loop for reentry to the atria and AV node (gold arrows). Because in both of these cases the His Purkinje system is still utilized, there is a narrow QRS complex.

administration, followed by a discussion with the patient that he or she might have an uncomfortable sensation in the chest, shortness of breath, and a sense of panic, which are all commonly encountered side effects. The first dose is 6 mg given by fast IV push, and, if unsuccessful, followed by 12 mg. The speed at which this is administered is important due to adenosine's short half-life of less than 10 seconds. If this fails to establish a sinus rhythm, then synchronized cardioversion can be considered. In VF and pVT, unsynchronized cardioversion is done. If unsynchronized

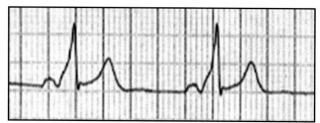

Figure 4-11. Example of WPW with a short PR interval (<0.12 milliseconds) and a delta wave secondary to an accessory pathway.

cardioversion is done in a patient with a regular rhythm SVT, the shock could occur during the vulnerable period of the conduction cycle related to commotio cordis. This could result in a patient deteriorating into VT or VF. In a stable patient with SVT, calcium channel or beta blockers can also be considered; however, these are not first-line therapy.

Wolff-Parkinson-White Syndrome

WPW syndrome, one form of ventricular pre-excitation, is a well-known condition that is associated with an accessory pathway connecting the atria and ventricles (see Figure 4-10b). Compared to normal AV nodal conduction, ventricular conduction via the accessory pathway excites the ventricular myocardium earlier, but in a more disorganized manner than impulses using the His-Purkinje system. This is because electrical impulses do not have to pass through the AV node, which has a short pause before continuing to the ventricles, and do not use the His-Purkinje system. Due to ventricular depolarization occurring simultaneously through both the normal pathway and the accessory pathway, a slightly widened QRS complex can be observed, with a short PR interval and slurring of the R wave on EKG known as a *delta wave* (Figure 4-11).[7,78] However, it is also possible for these individuals to have a normal EKG at rest due to their heart not using the accessory pathway, with abnormalities identified only with tachycardia during activity.[79]

In patients with WPW syndrome who are suffering from a reentrant tachycardia, there are 2 subtypes: orthodromic (retrograde) and antidromic (anterograde). In orthodromic AVRT, conduction travels through the AV node in the usual direction and back up the accessory pathway, and thus a normal QRS complex with no delta wave is observed (see Figure 4-10B). This narrow regular QRS complex tachycardia in a patient with a known history of WPW syndrome should be treated like paroxysmal SVT.

In contrast, antidromic AVRT involves conduction down the accessory pathway and travels retrograde up

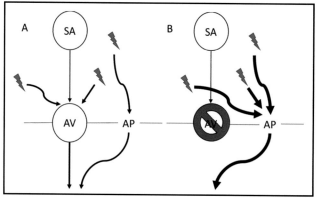

Figure 4-12. (A) schematic representation of a patient with atrial fibrillation/flutter using the accessory pathway in WPW. (B) When an AV nodal blocking agent is used in this patient, the atrial electrical impulses follow the path of least resistance (AP), thus creating the irregular WCT. Abbreviations: SA, SA node; AV, AV node; AP, accessory pathway.

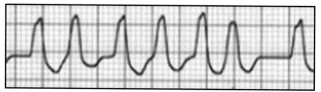

Figure 4-13. Example of a WCT with an irregular rhythm from atrial fibrillation/flutter in a patient with WPW.

the AV node.[7] This subtype is associated with a WCT due to the ventricular depolarization occurring outside of the His-Purkinje system. In these cases, AV nodal blocking agents, such as adenosine, beta blockers, and certain calcium-channel blockers, should be used with caution to avoid further preference for accessory pathway conduction (Figure 4-12). These drugs can cause fatal arrhythmias, especially in those with atrial fibrillation or flutter.[7,78] Accessory pathways, with shorter refractory periods compared to the AV node, allow for faster ventricular rates than seen with AV nodal conduction. A WCT with rates up to 300 beats per minute can be observed in those with atrial fibrillation or flutter (Figure 4-13). Even in young, healthy patients, ventricular conduction at this rate can precipitate quickly to VF and cardiac arrest. Use of AV nodal blocking agents in these patients allows for further hemodynamic compromise due to the increasing rate of the WCT. This WCT should be treated with procainamide, a class IA antiarrhythmic that slows conduction down the accessory pathway, or cardioversion, depending on whether the patient is hemodynamically stable or unstable, respectively.[7]

CHAPTER SUMMARY

- SCA should be assumed in any athlete with sudden collapse.
- SCD is more common in male athletes and is commonly seen in basketball and football players.
- An EKG may be the best screening tool currently available to detect predisposition to SCA, but its sensitivity and specificity are suboptimal.
- Athletes can have physiologic EKG changes related to intense exercise and conditioning. These should be differentiated from pathologic etiologies.
- A structurally normal heart is the most common finding in younger individuals with SCD, whereas coronary artery disease is most common in those greater than 35 years of age.
- Non-cardiac causes of SCA should always be considered.
- HCM in most individuals causes asymmetric thickening of the ventricular septum. This changes the physiology of the heart, causing exertional symptoms and possible syncope.
- ARVC causes replacement of normal heart tissue with adipose and fibrous tissue, disrupting the heart's intrinsic electrical activity, leading to fatal arrhythmias.
- WPW syndrome involves conduction through an accessory pathway connecting the atria and ventricles. This can present as a regular narrow QRS complex tachycardia and should be treated similarly to AVNRT. An irregular or wide QRS complex tachycardia in an individual with WPW syndrome should be treated with procainamide in a stable patient or synchronized cardioversion in an unstable patient.
- In many patients with conditions predisposing them to fatal arrhythmias, the first sign or symptom is SCA.
- Commotio cordis occurs when a blunt impact occurs over the chest wall during cardiac repolarization. It is treated like any other type of SCA.
- Time to defibrillation is the most important determinant of survival from SCA with VF, with a goal to defibrillation of less than 3 to 5 minutes.
- SCA with PEA or asystole should be treated with high-quality chest compressions and advanced cardiac life support.
- School-based programs that train individuals in CPR and the proper use of AEDs have helped improve the survival rate of SCA.
- EAPs should be implemented and continually reviewed to ensure prompt care of an athlete with SCA.

CHAPTER REVIEW QUESTIONS

1. A 14-year-old male athlete recently had his school sports physical. He has no history of syncopal events and no family history of SCD. His mother is concerned because in the past she was told he had a slow heart rate; however, he has never had any symptoms. His EKG shows a sinus bradycardia at 50 beats per minute, with a first-degree AV block. What is the next step?
   a) no further workup necessary
   b) repeat EKG in 1 month
   c) refer to a cardiologist
   d) obtain an EKG in mother

2. A 16-year-old softball player is stung by a bee. As she returns to the dugout, she is noted to be very sweaty and short of breath, then she collapses. She stops breathing and has no pulse. Aside from CPR, what is the most important next step?
   a) retrieving the AED
   b) administering epinephrine
   c) cooling the patient down with ice packs
   d) administering oxygen by non-rebreather mask

3. A baseball pitcher is hit in the chest with a line drive and immediately loses consciousness and stops breathing. What is the best management of this patient?
   a) do not perform CPR. as suspected rib fracture may cause further injury
   b) perform CPR, but there is no need to use an AED
   c) perform CPR and use an AED as soon as available
   d) administer oxygen and call for EMS to place the pitcher on a cardiac monitor

4. An autopsy is done on a 37-year-old male who suffered a SCD while starting a training regimen. What is most likely to be found as the etiology of his death?
   a) hypertrophic cardiomyopathy
   b) brugada syndrome
   c) coronary artery disease
   d) anomalous coronary artery

5. A 21-year-old female collapsed suddenly during a soccer game. Resuscitation efforts were unsuccessful. What is the most likely finding on autopsy?
   a) hypertrophic cardiomyopathy
   b) structurally normal heart
   c) coronary artery disease
   d) Wolff-Parkinson-White syndrome

ANSWERS

1. a
2. b
3. c
4. c
5. b

REFERENCES

1. Harmon KG, Zigman M, Drezner JA. The effectiveness of screening history, physical exam, and ECG to detect potentially lethal cardiac disorders in athletes: a systematic review/meta-analysis. *J Electrocardiol.* 2015;48(3):329-38. doi:10.1016/j.jelectrocard.2015.02.001.

2. Harmon K, Asif I, Ellenbogen R, et al. The incidence of sudden cardiac arrest and death in United States high school athletes. *Br J Sports Med.* 2014;48:605.

3. de Noronha SV, Sharma S, Papadakis M, Desai S, Whyte G, Sheppard MN. Aetiology of sudden cardiac death in athletes in the United Kingdom: a pathological study. *Heart.* 2009;95(17):1409-14. doi:10.1136/hrt.2009.168369.

4. Drezner JA, Sharma S, Baggish A, et al. International criteria for electrocardiographic interpretation in athletes: consensus statement. *Br J Sports Med.* 2017;51(9):704-731. doi:10.1136/bjsports-2016-097331.

5. Drezner JA, Ackerman MJ, Anderson J, et al. Electrocardiographic interpretation in athletes: the 'Seattle criteria'. *Br J Sports Med.* 2013;47(3):122-4. doi:10.1136/bjsports-2012-092067.

6. Prior DL, La Gerche A. The athlete's heart. *Heart.* 2012;98(12):947-55. doi:10.1136/heartjnl-2011-301329.

7. Lilly, Leonard S. *Pathophysiology of Heart Disease: A Collaborative Project of Medical Students and Faculty.* Baltimore, MD: Wolters Kluwer/Lippincott Williams and Wilkins, 2011.

8. Kramer E, Dvorak J, Kloeck W. Review of the management of sudden cardiac arrest on the football field. *Br J Sports Med.* 2010;44(8):540-5. doi:10.1136/bjsm.2010.074526.

9. Asif IM, Harmon KG. Incidence and etiology of sudden cardiac death: new updates for athletic departments. *Sports Health.* 2017;9(3):268-279. doi:10.1177/1941738117694153.

10. Wolfson AB. *Harwood-Nuss Clinical Practice of Emergency Medicine.* Philadelphia, PA: Wolters Kluwer; 2015.

11. Marijon E, Tafflet M, Celermajer DS, et al. Sports-related sudden death in the general population. *Circulation.* 2011;124(6):672-681. doi:10.1161/circulationaha.110.008979.

12. Harmon KG, Asif IM, Klossner D, Drezner JA. Incidence of sudden cardiac death in National Collegiate Athletic Association athletes. *Circulation.* 2011;123(15):1594-1600. doi:10.1161/circulationaha.110.004622.

13. Harmon KG, Asif IM, Maleszewski JJ. Incidence and etiology of sudden cardiac arrest and death in high school athletes in the United States. *Mayo Clin Proc.* 2016;91(11):1493-1502. doi:10.1016/j.mayocp.2016.07.021.

14. Drezner JA, Toresdahl BG, Rao AL, Huszti E, Harmon KG. Outcomes from sudden cardiac arrest in US high schools: a 2-year prospective study from the National Registry for AED Use in Sports. *Br J Sports Med.* 2013;47(18):1179-8113. doi:10.1136/bjsports-2013-092786.

15. Link MS. Clinical practice. Evaluation and initial treatment of supraventricular tachycardia. *N Engl J Med.* 2012;367(15):1438-48. doi:10.1056/NEJMcp1111259.

16. Webner D, DuPrey KM, Drezner JA, Cronholm P, Roberts WO. Sudden cardiac arrest and death in United States marathons. *Med Sci Sports Exerc.* 2012;44(10):1843-1845. doi:10.1249/MSS.0b013e318258b59a.

17. Landry CH, Allan KS, Connelly KA, et al. Sudden cardiac arrest during participation in competitive sports. *N Engl J Med.* 2017;377(20):1943-1953. doi:10.1056/NEJMoa1615710.

18. Harmon KG, Drezner JA, Maleszewski JJ, et al. Pathogeneses of sudden cardiac death in national collegiate athletic association athletes. *Circ Arrhythm Electrophysiol.* 2014;7(2):198-204. doi:10.1161/CIRCEP.113.001376.

19. Peterson DF, Siebert DM, Kucera KL, et al. Etiology of sudden cardiac arrest and death in us competitive athletes: a 2-year prospective surveillance study. *Clin J Sport Med.* 2018 [Epub ahead of print]. doi:10.1097/JSM.0000000000000598.

20. Chandra N, Bastiaenen R, Papadakis M, Sharma S. Sudden cardiac death in young athletes: practical challenges and diagnostic dilemmas. *J Am Coll Cardiol.* 2013;61(10):1027-40. doi:10.1016/j.jacc.2012.08.1032.

21. Maron BJ, Doerer JJ, Haas TS, Tierney DM, Mueller FO. Sudden deaths in young competitive athletes: analysis of 1866 deaths in the United States, 1980-2006. *Circulation.* 2009;119(8):1085-1092. doi:10.1161/circulationaha.108.804617.

22. Fineschi V, Riezzo I, Centini F, et al. Sudden cardiac death during anabolic steroid abuse: morphologic and toxicologic findings in two fatal cases of bodybuilders. *Int J Legal Med.* 2007;121(1):48-53.

23. Dickerman RD, Schaller F, Prather I, McConathy WJ. Sudden cardiac death in a 20-year-old bodybuilder using anabolic steroids. *Cardiology.* 1995;86(2):172-173.

24. Lichtenfeld J, Deal BJ, Crawford S. Sudden cardiac arrest following ventricular fibrillation attributed to anabolic steroid use in an adolescent. *Cardiol Young.* 2016;26(5):996-998. doi:10.1017/S104795111600007X.

25. Eckart RE, Shry EA, Burke AP, et al. Sudden death in young adults: an autopsy-based series of a population undergoing active surveillance. *J Am Coll Cardiol.* 2011;58(12):1254-1261. doi:10.1016/j.jacc.2011.01.049.

26. Pigozzi F, Rizzo M. Sudden death in competitive athletes. *Clin Sports Med.* 2008;27(1):153-181, ix. doi:10.1016/j.csm.2007.09.004.

27. Mittleman MA, Maclure M, Tofler GH, Sherwood JB, Goldberg RJ, Muller JE. Triggering of acute myocardial infarction by heavy physical exertion. Protection against triggering by regular exertion. Determinants of myocardial infarction onset study investigators. *N Engl J Med.* 1993;329(23):1677-1683.

28. Houston BA, Stevens GR. Hypertrophic Cardiomyopathy: A Review. *Clin Med Insights Cardiol.* 2014;8(Suppl 1):53-65. doi:10.4137/CMC.S15717.

29. Tabib A, Loire R, Chalabreysse L, et al. Circumstances of death and gross and microscopic observations in a series of 200 cases of sudden death associated with arrhythmogenic right ventricular cardiomyopathy and/or dysplasia. *Circulation.* 2003;108(24):3000-3005.

30. Trivedi A, Knight BP. ICD therapy for primary prevention in hypertrophic cardiomyopathy. *Arrhythm Electrophysiol Rev.* 2016;5(3):188-196. doi:10.15420/aer.2016:30:2.

31. Sen-Chowdhry S, Lowe MD, Sporton SC, McKenna WJ. Arrhythmogenic right ventricular cardiomyopathy: clinical presentation, diagnosis, and management. *Am J Med.* 2004;117(9):685-695.

32. Dalal D, Nasir K, Bomma C, et al. Arrhythmogenic right ventricular dysplasia: a United States experience. *Circulation.* 2005;112(25):3823-3832.

33. Gemayel C, Pelliccia A, Thompson PD. Arrhythmogenic right ventricular cardiomyopathy. *J Am Coll Cardiol.* 2001;38(7):1773-1781.

34. Corrado D, Basso C, Rizzoli G, Schiavon M, Thiene G. Does sports activity enhance the risk of sudden death in adolescents and young adults? *J Am Coll Cardiol.* 2003;42(11):1959-1963.

35. Walker J, Calkins H, Nazarian S. Evaluation of cardiac arrhythmia among athletes. *Am J Med.* 2010;123(12):1075-1081. doi:10.1016/j.amjmed.2010.05.008.

36. Modell SM, Lehmann MH. The long QT syndrome family of cardiac ion channelopathies: a HuGE review. *Genet Med.* 2006;8(3):143-155.

37. Fazio G, Vernuccio F, Grutta G, Re GL. Drugs to be avoided in patients with long QT syndrome: focus on the anaesthesiological management. *World J Cardiol.* 2013;5(4):87-93. doi:10.4330/wjc.v5.i4.87.

38. Basavarajaiah S, Wilson M, Whyte G, Shah A, Behr E, Sharma S. Prevalence and significance of an isolated long QT interval in elite athletes. *Eur Heart J.* 2007;28(23):2944-2949.

39. Rudic B, Schimpf R, Borggrefe M. Short QT syndrome—review of diagnosis and treatment. *Arrhythm Electrophysiol Review.* 2014;3(2):76-79. doi:10.15420/aer.2014.3.2.76.

40. Pavão MLRC, Ono VC, Arfelli E, Simões MV, Marin Neto JA, Schmidt A. Sudden cardiac death and short QT syndrome. *Arq Bras Cardiol.* 2014;103(3):e37-e40. doi:10.5935/abc.20140133.

41. Vohra J, Rajagopalan S; CSANZ Genetics Council Writing Group. Update on the diagnosis and management of Brugada syndrome. *Heart Lung Circ.* 2015;24(12):1141-1148. doi:10.1016/j.hlc.2015.07.020.

42. Antzelevitch C, Brugada P, Borggrefe M, et al. Brugada syndrome: report of the second consensus conference: endorsed by the Heart Rhythm Society and the European Heart Rhythm Association. *Circulation.* 2005;111(5):659-670.

43. Willich SN, Lewis M, Löwel H, Arntz HR, Schubert F, Schröder R. Physical exertion as a trigger of acute myocardial infarction. Triggers and mechanisms of myocardial infarction study group. *N Engl J Med.* 1993;329(23):1684-1690.

44. Drezner JA, Courson RW, Roberts WO, et al. Inter Association Task Force recommendations on emergency preparedness and management of sudden cardiac arrest in high school and college athletic programs: a consensus statement. *Prehosp Emerg Care.* 2007;11(3):253-271.

45. Farrokhian AR. Commotio cordis and Contusio cordis: possible causes of trauma-related cardiac death. *Arch Trauma Res.* 2016;5(4):e41482. doi:10.5812/atr.41482.

46. Link MS, Maron BJ, VanderBrink BA, et al. Impact directly over the cardiac silhouette is necessary to produce ventricular fibrillation in an experimental model of commotio cordis. *J Am Coll Cardiol.* 2001;37(2):649-654.

47. Kalin J, Madias C, Alsheikh-Ali AA, Link MS. Reduced diameter spheres increases the risk of chest blow-induced ventricular fibrillation (commotio cordis). *Heart Rhythm.* 2011; 8(10):1578-81. doi:10.1016/j.hrthm.2011.05.009.

48. Madias C, Maron BJ, Dau N, Estes NAM 3rd, Bir C, Link MS. Size as an important determinant of chest blow-induced Commotio cordis. *Med Sci Sports Exerc.* 2018; 50(9): 1767-1771. doi:10.1249/MSS.0000000000001630.

49. Weinstock J, Maron BJ, Song C, Mane PP, Estes NA 3rd, Link MS. Failure of commercially available chest wall protectors to prevent sudden cardiac death induced by chest wall blows in an experimental model of commotio cordis. *Pediatrics.* 2006; 117(4):e656-662.

50. Link MS, Estes NA 3rd, Maron BJ et al. Eligibility and disqualification recommendations for competitive athletes with cardiovascular abnormalities: task force 13: commotio cordis: a scientific statement from the American Heart Association and American College of Cardiology. *Circulation.* 2015; 132(22):e339-e342. doi:10.1161/CIR.0000000000000249.

51. Brennan FH Jr, Stenzler B, Oriscello R. Diagnosis and management of myocarditis in athletes. *Curr Sports Med Rep.* 2003 Apr;2(2):65-71. Review. PubMed PMID: 12831661.

52. Caforio AL, Pankuweit S, Arbustini E, et al. Current state of knowledge on aetiology, diagnosis, management, and therapy of myocarditis: a position statement of the European Society of Cardiology Working Group on Myocardial and Pericardial Diseases, *Eur Heart J.* 2013;34(33):2636-2648. doi:10.1093/eurheartj/eht210.

53. Khandaker MH, Espinosa RE, Nishimura RA, et al. Pericardial disease: diagnosis and management. *Mayo Clin Proc.* 2010;85(6):572-593. doi:10.4065/mcp.2010.0046.

54. Seidenberg PH, Haynes J. Pericarditis: diagnosis, management, and return to play. *Curr Sports Med Rep.* 2006;5(2):74-79.

55. 2018 Physical Activity Guidelines Advisory Committee. Scientific Report. Washington, DC: US Department of Health and Human Services, 2018.

56. Albert CM, Mittleman MA, Chae CU, Lee IM, Hennekens CH, Manson JE. Triggering of sudden death from cardiac causes by vigorous exertion. *N Engl J Med.* 2000;343(19):1355-61.

57. Willich SN, Lewis M, Löwel H, Arntz HR, Schubert F, Schröder R. Physical exertion as a trigger of acute myocardial infarction. *N Engl J Med.* 1993;329(23):1684-1690.

58. Neilan TG, Januzzi JL, Lee-Lewandrowski E, et al. Myocardial injury and ventricular dysfunction related to training levels among nonelite participants in the Boston marathon. *Circulation.* 2006; 114(22):2325-33.

59. Panhuyzen-Goedkoop NM, Wellens HJ, Piek JJ. Early recognition of sudden cardiac arrest in athletes during sports activity. *Neth Heart J.* 2018;26(1):21-25. doi:10.1007/s12471-017-1061-5.

60. Terry GC, Kyle JM, Ellis JM Jr, Cantwell J, Courson R, Medlin R. Sudden cardiac arrest in athletic medicine. *J Athl Train.* 2001;36(2):205-209.

61. Bækgaard JS, Viereck S, Møller TP, Ersbøll AK, Lippert F, Folke F. The effects of public access defibrillation on survival after out-of-hospital cardiac arrest: a systematic review of observational studies. *Circulation.* 2017; 136(10):954-965. doi:10.1161/circulationaha.117.029067.

62. Drezner JA, Chun JS, Harmon KG, Derminer L. Survival trends in the United States following exercise-related sudden cardiac arrest in the youth: 2000-2006. *Heart Rhythm.* 2008; 5(6):794-9. doi:10.1016/j.hrthm.2008.03.001.

63. Panchal AR, Berg MD, Kudenchuk PJ, et al. 2018 American Heart association focused update on advanced cardiovascular life suport use of antiarrhythmic drugs during and immediately after cardiac arrest. *Circulation.* 2018;138:e740-749. doi:10.1161/CIR.0000000000000613.

64. Eberle B, Dick WF, Schneider T, Wisser G, Doetsch S, Tzanova I. Checking the carotid pulse check: diagnostic accuracy of first responders in patients with and without a pulse. *Resuscitation.* 1996;33(2):107-116.

65. Ruppert M, Reith MW, Widmann JH, et al. Checking for breathing: evaluation of the diagnostic capability of emergency medical services personnel, physicians, medical students, and medical laypersons. *Ann Emerg Med.* 1999;34(6):720-729.

66. Lapostolle F, Le Toumelin P, Agostinucci JM, Catineau J, Adnet F. Basic cardiac life support providers checking the carotid pulse: performance, degree of conviction, and influencing factors. *Acad Emerg Med.* 2004;11(8):878-880.

67. Kleinman ME, Brennan EE, Goldberger ZD, et al. 2015 American Heart Association guidelines update for cardiopulmonary resuscitation and emergency cardiovascular care, part 5: adult basic life support and cardiopulmonary resuscitation quality: *Circulation.* 2015;132(18 Suppl 2):S414-35. doi:10.1161/CIR.0000000000000259.

68. Kramer EB, Botha M, Drezner J, Abdelrahman Y, Dvorak J. Practical management of sudden cardiac arrest on the football field. *Br J Sports Med.* 2012; 46(16):1094-1096. doi:10.1136/bjsports-2012-091376.

69. Drezner JA. Preparing for sudden cardiac arrest—the essential role of automated external defibrillators in athletic medicine: a critical review. *Br J Sports Med.* 2009;43(9):702-707. doi:10.1136/bjsm.2008.054890.

70. Hazinski MF, Markenson D, Neish S, et al. Response to cardiac arrest and selected life-threatening medical emergencies: the medical emergency response plan for schools: A statement for healthcare providers, policymakers, school administrators, and community leaders. *Circulation.* 2004;109(2):278-291.

71. Berg RA, Kern KB, Sanders AB, Otto CW, Hilwig RW, Ewy GA. Bystander cardiopulmonary resuscitation. Is ventilation necessary? *Circulation.* 1993;88(4 Pt 1):1907-1915.

72. Berg RA, Sanders AB, Kern KB, et al. Adverse hemodynamic effects of interrupting chest compressions for rescue breathing during cardiopulmonary resuscitation for ventricular fibrillation cardiac arrest. *Circulation.* 2001;104(20):2465-2470.

73. Bohm K, Rosenqvist M, Herlitz J, Hollenberg J, Svensson L. Survival is similar after standard treatment and chest compression only in out-of-hospital bystander cardiopulmonary resuscitation. *Circulation.* 2007; 116(25):2908-2912.

74. Benjamin EJ, Blaha MJ, Chiuve SE, et al. Heart disease and stroke statistics—2017 update: a report from the American Heart Association. *Circulation.* 2017;135(10):e146-e603. doi:10.1161/CIR.0000000000000485.

75. Becker LB, Ostrander MP, Barrett J, Kondos GT. Outcome of CPR in a large metropolitan area—where are the survivors? *Ann Emerg Med.* 1991 Apr;20(4):355-361.

76. Drezner JA, Rao AL, Heistand J, Bloomingdale MK, Harmon KG. Effectiveness of emergency response planning for sudden cardiac arrest in United States high schools with automated external defibrillators. *Circulation.* 2009; 120(6):518-525. doi:10.1161/circulationaha.109.855890.

77. Waninger KN, Goodbred A, Vanic K, et al. Adequate performance of cardiopulmonary resuscitation techniques during simulated cardiac arrest over and under protective equipment in football. *Clin J Sport Med.* 2014;24(4):280-3. doi:10.1097/JSM.0000000000000022.

78. ECC Committee, Subcommittees and Task Forces of the American Heart Association. 2005 American Heart Association guidelines for cardiopulmonary resuscitation and emergency cardiovascular care. *Circulation.* 2005;112(24 Suppl):IV1-203.

79. Drezner JA, Peterson DF, Siebert DM, et al. Survival after exercise-related sudden cardiac arrest in young athletes: can we do better? *Sports Health.* 2019; 11(1):91-98. doi:10.1177/1941738118799084.

5

Endocrine Emergencies

John Murphy, DO; Robert O. Blanc, MS, LAT, ATC, EMT-P; and James Medure

CHAPTER KEY WORDS

- Adrenal system
- Hypothalamus
- Pituitary

CHAPTER SCENARIO

You are called to the wrestling room where practice has been in progress for 25 minutes. Upon arriving, you are told that one of the wrestlers has been acting "different" and "not himself." He is conscious, but anxious and agitated. His speech is mildly slurred, and he feels fatigued. You know the athlete, who has been cutting weight recently, has diabetes mellitus.

SCENARIO RESOLUTION

You question the athlete regarding his dietary habits for the day and learn that because he is trying to cut weight, he has not had anything substantial to eat today. You immediately measure his blood glucose level and get a reading of 64 mg/dL. You administer a sugar packet to him and check his vital signs. All vitals are within normal limits, and he states he feels better after just a few minutes. After 15 minutes, you recheck his blood glucose level and get a reading of 78 mg/dL. He then eats a carbohydrate snack bar, and after 15 more minutes, his blood glucose level is 112 mg/dL. The athlete is cleared to return to practice, with repeat glucose checks every 15 to 20 minutes.

INTRODUCTION

Every day our body responds nearly instantaneously via the central and peripheral nervous system (CNS and PNS); some of these are conscious and some are subconsciously controlled. This communication is evident in every action we make, but it is also occurring without our realization. The CNS and PNS comprise a collection of specialized cells called *neurons* that connect our brain to our organs and tissues. The CNS communicates with the hypothalamus in the brain to stimulate certain hormones to be produced. Hormones are regulatory substances generated in specific organs in the body and transported via blood. Every function we perform requires a homeostatic balance to ensure proper body temperature, blood sugar, heart rate, and metabolism. Thanks to the endocrine system, this happens without any conscious effort.

Specifically, the hypothalamus (which interacts with the CNS) and pituitary are responsible for the initial hormones for growth, metabolism, and reproduction, which then stimulate endocrine organs that include the thyroid and adrenal glands (or suprarenal glands, which are found above the kidneys).[1] The thyroid gland and adrenal glands then respond to the input from the pituitary as to how much thyroid hormone or cortisol, respectively, to produce.[1] The pancreas is both an endocrine and exocrine organ that is responsible for maintaining proper blood sugar levels and

Feld F., Gorse KM, Blanc RO
Non-Orthopedic Emergency Care in Athletics (pp 35-41).
© 2020 Taylor & Francis Group.

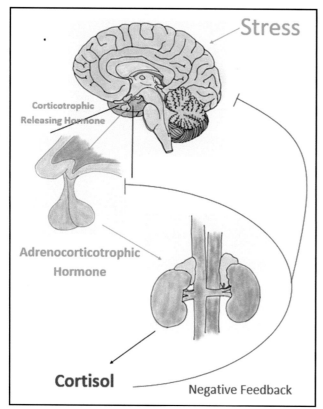

Figure 5-1. Negative feedback to the hypothalamus and pituitary glands.

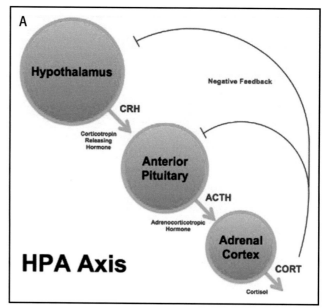

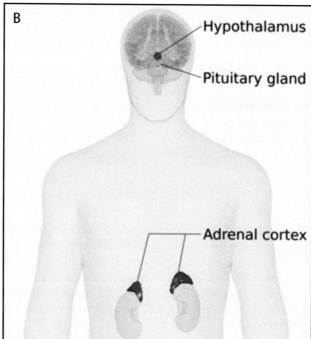

Figures 5-2A and 5-2B. HPA axis provides hormone production control.

preventing life-threatening conditions such as diabetic ketoacidosis. With improved care and early recognition, these conditions can either be prevented before they occur or before they become life-threatening.

The hypothalamic–pituitary–adrenal axis involves a complex group of direct influences and feedback mechanisms among 3 organs: the hypothalamus, the pituitary gland (below the thalamus), and the adrenal (or suprarenal) glands. The hypothalamus connects the neurological system to the endocrine system with neuroendocrine cells that generate hormones (eg, the corticotropin-releasing hormone) to communicate with the pituitary gland to secrete more or less hormones. In response, the pituitary gland generates and secretes stimulating hormones, such as adrenocorticotropic hormone, that travel through the blood to the adrenal cortex to signal rapid production of corticosteroids, including cortisol. The production of cortisol in the adrenal gland will then provide negative feedback to the hypothalamus and pituitary to inhibit production of corticotropin-releasing hormone and adrenocorticotropic hormone, respectively, to prevent overproduction of hormones (Figure 5-1).[1]

This is an overview of how the entire hypothalamic–pituitary–adrenal axis works to provide our bodies with the appropriate levels of hormones in a given situation. The hypothalamic–pituitary axis specifically generates hormones responsible for metabolism, reproduction, and growth. The adrenal gland is responsible for stress hormones and sex hormones, as well as for assisting with blood pressure regulation. These hormones do not perform these tasks alone; they simply aid the homeostasis to maintain proper function of their respective organs (Figure 5-2).[1,2]

Thyroid Gland

The thyroid gland is a bilobed gland that sits anterior to the trachea in the neck. The thyroid gland is part of its own neuroendocrine hypothalamic–pituitary axis system referred to as the *hypothalamic–pituitary–thyroid axis*. The hypothalamus produces thyrotropin-releasing hormone when circulating thyroid levels are low, which stimulates the anterior pituitary to generate the thyroid-stimulating hormone (TSH), which then stimulates the thyroid gland to produce more thyroid hormone.[1] Similar to the adrenal gland, the appropriate levels of thyroid in the blood act as negative feedback to the hypothalamus to prevent it from generating too much thyrotropin-releasing hormone. Thyroid hormone specifically helps regulate metabolism and growth. It does so with the help of the mineral iodine, which is obtained from our diet; that is why salt is generally iodized. Without proper amounts of iodine in our diet, we run the risk of hypothyroidism (Figure 5-3).[1]

Hyperthyroidism

Hyperthyroidism is a form of thyrotoxicosis, which is excessive thyroid hormone of any kind. Hyperthyroidism results from an increased production of T3 and/or T4 thyroid hormones produced by the thyroid gland.[1] There is a wide range of severity of hyperthyroidism, and the most severe case, *thyroid storm*, results in confusion, an irregular heartbeat, vomiting, diarrhea, and elevated core body temperature. Thyroid storm is a true medical emergency that can result in death in up to 50% of patients, even if it is identified and treated rapidly.

Causes of hyperthyroidism include Graves' disease (50% to 80%), thyroid adenoma, multinodular goiter, inflammation of the thyroid gland, endogenous iodine consumption, and excessive synthetic iodine ingestion (for treatment of hypothyroidism). Signs and symptoms include nervousness, tremors, tachycardia, palpitations, irritability, heat intolerance, muscle weakness, diarrhea, enlarged thyroid, weight loss, sleeping difficulty, and possibly an enlarging neck mass called a *goiter*.[1,2] These are often vague, and this diagnosis should be considered frequently, as it may be asymptomatic at the time of diagnosis. Diagnosis of hyperthyroidism is identified with blood tests that include a low TSH and elevated T3 and/or T4 hormones. The appropriate provider should perform further testing to identify the cause of the hyperthyroidism. Treatment depends on the severity, symptoms, and blood levels of T3 and/or T4, but it can include beta blockers, corticosteroids, radioactive ablation, and surgery to remove the thyroid gland.[1,2]

Hypothyroidism

On the other hand, hypothyroidism results from an underproduction of thyroid hormone by the thyroid gland. Symptoms may include fatigue, weight gain, cold intolerance, constipation, and depression. Just like hyperthyroidism, this too may result in a goiter. This condition is particularly concerning during pregnancy, as it can result in cretinism, with developmental and growth delays in the fetus. The most extreme form of hypothyroidism is *myxedema coma*, a life-threatening condition that causes low

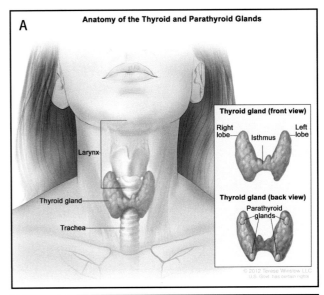

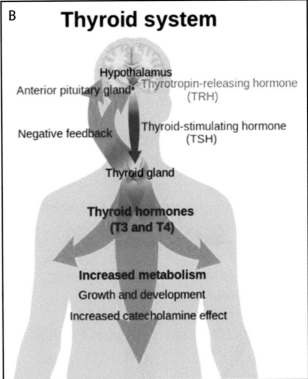

Figures 5-3A and 5-3B. Production of thyroid hormones maintains metabolism and growth. (5-3A Illustration by Terese Winslow, 2012)

body temperature without compensatory shivering, lethargy, confusion, bradycardia, and bradypnea.[3]

Around the world, the most common cause of hypothyroidism is lack of iodine. In more developed countries, where adequate iodine is consumed in part from iodized salt, the most common cause of hypothyroidism is Hashimoto's thyroiditis. This is an autoimmune condition, called *chronic lymphocytic thyroiditis*, in which the patient's own lymphocytes generate antibodies to thyroid gland cells, which eventually destroys the thyroid gland.[3] Other causes include thyroid surgery, radioactive ablation of

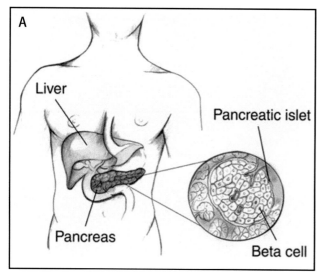

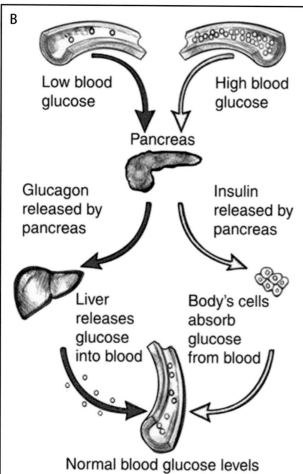

Figures 5-4A and 5-4B. Insulin and glucagon production control blood glucose levels.

thyroid gland, medications, or injury to the hypothalamus or pituitary. Similar to hyperthyroidism, hypothyroidism is also diagnosed with bloodwork. Positive results, however, will be the opposite, with an elevated TSH and low T3 and/ or T4 levels. Treatment often begins with synthetic thyroid

hormone replacement such as levothyroxine. Levels of TSH are then monitored to evaluate for proper dosage amount.[1,2]

Diabetes

The pancreas is a mixed-function organ that has both endocrine and exocrine (which secretes digestive juices) components. It is located in the upper left quadrant of the stomach (Figure 5-4A). It functions in digestion by secreting transglutaminase pancreatic digestive enzymes to break down food and better absorb nutrients in the small intestine, as well as bicarbonate to neutralize the acidity of the chyme (partially digested food leaving the stomach) prior to its reaching the small intestine.[4] It also functions as an endocrine organ by producing hormones such as insulin and glucagon. These hormones are secreted directly into the blood. Within the pancreas, clusters of cells called *islets of Langerhans* contain both alpha and beta cells. These cells secrete glucagon and insulin, respectively; both are critical to glucose metabolism and homeostasis. Glucagon functions by increasing blood glucose, and insulin functions by decreasing blood glucose. (Figure 5-4B).[4]

Diabetes mellitus (commonly referred to as *diabetes*, but not to be confused with diabetes insipidus) is a metabolic disorder of glucose metabolism. It results in either an elevation or a reduction in blood sugar. Generally speaking, diabetes falls into the following 2 categories[4]:

1. Type I: the lack of insulin production is believed to be the result of the islets of Langerhans being destroyed by an autoimmune condition.

2. Type II: resistance to insulin is the most common type.

Insulin is a peptide hormone made in the pancreatic beta cells. Its main function is to bring glucose from the bloodstream into cells. For this reason, it is considered the body's main anabolic hormone. Beta cells respond to blood sugar levels, and when the levels rise above a certain threshold, they secrete insulin.[4]

The exact cause of a lack of insulin production by the pancreas is not known, but it is believed to be due an autoimmune disease. The beta cells, which produce insulin, are attacked and destroyed by the body's own immune system, often after a viral infection. Type I diabetes more commonly occurs in children and young adults.

The cause of type II diabetes is not well understood, but is believed to be associated with obesity, poor dietary habits, and a sedentary lifestyle.[5,6]

When insulin ceases to be produced, or the cells become resistant to the insulin, blood glucose levels rise. The body will attempt to lower the sugar levels by eliminating it through the urine. Dehydration occurs due to excessive urination, or *polyuria*, as water follows the sugar. As dehydration increases, thirst, or *polydipsia*, will increase. Polyuria and polydipsia are early signs of type I diabetes. Patients will more commonly present with these signs and symptoms, which often begin occurring gradually over weeks, months, or even years. Some of the less commonly identified symptoms include weight loss, blurry vision, headaches, fatigue, and slow healing of wounds or injuries.[5,6,7]

As this continues, the blood sugar keeps rising, but the cells are still unable to use the glucose. The body will go into a starvation mode, which will cause an increase in the person's thirst and hunger, called *polyphagia*. Ketoacids are produced as the body attempts to break down fats and proteins as an alternate energy source. When ketoacids are present, dehydration occurs, along with rapid breathing and changes in mental status. Known as *ketoacidosis*, this can cause the patient to present with nausea, vomiting, sweet breath odor, abdominal pain, rapid deep breathing (ie, Kussmaul's respirations), and mental status changes or coma.[7]

Polyuria, polydipsia, and polyphagia may also occur in individuals with type II diabetes, but the mechanism by which they occur is slightly different. In the case of a type II diabetic, medications are available to stimulate insulin production, affect the liver's production of glucose, and decrease the body's ability to absorb sugar and resist insulin.[4]

When caring for individuals with diabetes, 2 emergent conditions may arise. In hypoglycemia, the blood glucose levels fall, usually due to too much insulin being administered without proper food intake. This causes cells to lack energy derived from sugar, which does not allow the cells to function properly. Because brain cells are sensitive to a decrease in sugar availability, a decrease in mental status may occur. Also, a person suffering from hypoglycemia may appear cool, clammy, and pale; may act abnormal, confused, anxious, and aggressive; and may complain of dizziness, headache, or visual changes. If allowed to progress, unconsciousness and seizures may follow. This is the most common in type I diabetes due to too much insulin being given; however, type II diabetes may also cause hypoglycemia, perhaps due to the individual's use of some medications or illness.[4,6,7]

When blood glucose levels become too high, hyperglycemia occurs. When cells do not or cannot use sugar, polyuria, polydipsia, and polyphagia ("the 3 Ps") occur. This may also be seen in a person with sepsis. In an effort to gain energy for cells, the body will break down proteins and fats. This produces ketoacids, which in turn increases acidosis and triggers dehydration. Ketoacidosis generally has a prolonged development over hours or even days. Ketoacidosis may present with abdominal pain, nausea, vomiting, confusion, rapid deep breathing, and, potentially, coma.[7]

Assessment

As with any evaluation, taking a thorough history is of utmost importance. In evaluating a patient with known diabetes, the history should include recent food intake, insulin dosage time and dosage, most recent blood glucose levels, and symptoms. In a confused or unconscious patient, an immediate blood glucose level should be obtained. This can be done with a glucometer, which should be readily available. Under normal conditions, a fasting blood glucose level should be between 60 and 100 mg/dL. This range may increase to 120 or 150 mg/dL after eating. A blood glucose level below 60 mg/dL may cause symptoms associated with hypoglycemia, including decreased mental function. If levels are above 250 mg/dL, hyperglycemia may occur, with symptoms that include the 3 Ps and altered mental status.[4,6,7,8]

Emergency Care

As in any emergency situation, proper preparation is the first step in successfully caring for a patient with diabetes suffering from insulin-related emergencies. This includes having an emergency action plan that is well-thought-out, communicated, and practiced. Immediate access to blood glucose monitoring equipment is essential. Be sure that test strips are current and the batteries are charged—having spare batteries on hand is important. Having urine test strips to measure ketones is also necessary.[6,7]

Preparation for a patient who is deemed to be hypoglycemic should include a glucagon injection kit, glucose tablets, and foods and beverages high in sugar, such as orange juice, non-diet soda, sugar packets, and candy.

If the patient becomes hyperglycemic, access to insulin is required. This may be administered via the patient's pump or by injection. All potential caregivers should know the proper use of the pump.

When a patient is hypoglycemic, with a blood glucose level less than 70 mg/dL, the following steps should be taken:

- Assess the level of consciousness and ability to safely swallow.
- If the person is unconscious or unresponsive, administer a glucagon injection and notify 911.
- If the person is conscious and able to swallow, have the patient take a drink or eat a piece of candy. After 10 to 15 minutes, repeat glucose testing and monitor mental status. Serial readings should be repeated every 15 minutes until the patient returns to baseline. Care should be taken not to overtreat the hypoglycemia. A blood glucose reading between 70 mg/dL and 99 mg/dL should be monitored closely. If the patient

is asymptomatic, provide a snack and recheck blood glucose level in 15 minutes. If the reading is greater than 100 mg/dL, the patient may return to activity. If the blood glucose level is greater than 250 mg/dL, the urine should be checked for ketones. If no ketones are present, the individual may exercise with caution. If ketones are present, activity should be halted until the person is asymptomatic, ketones are no longer present, and the blood glucose level is greater than 300 mg/dL.[4,6,7,8]

See Appendix 1 for a diabetic treatment algorithm.

Chapter Summary

Endocrine-related issues in an athletic population present special considerations concerning identification, treatment, and proper management. Although of concern, these endocrine conditions do not disqualify athletes from participation, but special precautions should be taken to ensure the athlete's health and well-being.

Hyperthyroidism is a medical emergency that is potentially fatal if untreated, and athletes of concern should complete proper blood tests, followed by an associated medication for management.[1,2] Hypothyroidism should also be confirmed using blood diagnostic tests to ensure diagnosis, and the athlete should receive the correct medication. Clinicians should be aware of concerning symptoms in both conditions and be aware of the medications athletes are taking for regulation of the thyroid gland.[3]

Type I diabetes, more common in younger populations, is the complete lack of insulin production, whereas type II diabetes, more common in sedentary individuals, is a resistance to insulin. In type I diabetes, ketoacidosis can occur from ketoacids that are produced to break down fats and proteins, coupled with dehydration caused by polyuria. These events can also occur in type II diabetes; however, medication stimulates insulin production to allow the body to absorb sugar.

Hypoglycemia and hyperglycemia are emergent conditions that should be monitored in individuals with pre-existing knowledge of the condition. In hypoglycemia, when blood glucose levels drop due to excess insulin without proper dietary intake, the lack of energy in cells can cause altered mental status, and rapid management is imperative. In hyperglycemia, when blood glucose levels are elevated, ketones in the urine should immediately be assessed, and insulin should be administered.[5,6,7]

For proper care and management of diabetic episodes, food intake, insulin time and dosage, blood glucose levels,

and symptoms are vital information. Blood glucose less than 60 mg/dL could render the patient hypoglycemic, and levels above 250 mg/dL could render the patient hyperglycemic. If the patient is unresponsive, emergency services should be summoned. Management should include testing glucose levels and ketones while having access to glucagon injection kits, glucose tablets, or fast-acting consumable sugar products for hypoglycemic patients, and access to immediate insulin for hyperglycemic patients. If hypoglycemic, administer fast-acting sugar and reassess blood glucose levels every 10 to 15 minutes to prevent overcompensation. When levels fall between 70 and 99 mg/dL, monitor and provide glucose substitutes every 15 minutes until levels are greater than 100 mg/dL, when the athlete can return to monitored activity. If glucose levels are above 250 mg/dL, urine must be checked for ketones. If none are present, the athlete can return to activity with caution. If ketones are present, activity is halted until ketones are no longer present and glucose levels are below 250 mg/dL.[6]

Quick, accurate assessment, along with proper identification and management of endocrine-related episodes, can drastically affect treatment success. Prior knowledge of endocrine-related issues, as well as preparation for episodes, would allow proper treatment and provide patients with the highest level of care possible.

Chapter Review Questions

1. Describe the symptoms of a thyroid storm.
2. What condition can result from a lack of iodine?
3. Describe the difference between type I and type II diabetes.
4. What items should be readily available on the sidelines if an athlete has diabetes?

Answers

1. Confusion, irregular heartbeat, vomiting, diarrhea, and elevated core body temperature.
2. Hypothyroidism.
3. Type I is characterized by lack of insulin production. Type II is characterized by resistance to insulin.
4. Emergency action plan, glucometer, urine test strips, glucagon injection kit, glucose tablets, and foods and beverages high in sugar.

REFERENCES

1. Welt CK. Hypothalamic-pituitary axis. UpToDate. https://www.uptodate.com/contents/hypothalamic-pituitary-axis?search=hypothalamicpituitaryaxis&source=search_result&selectedTitle=1~150&usage_type=default&display_rank=1. Accessed November 15, 2018.

2. Kidd GS, Glass AR, Vigersky RA. The hypothalamic-pituitary-testicular axis in thyrotoxicosis. *J Clin Endocrinol Metab.* 1979;48(5):798-802.

3. Kwaku MP, Burman KD. Myxedema coma. *J Intensive Care Med.* 2007;22(4):224-231.

4. McCulloch, DK. Overview of medical care in adults with diabetes mellitus. UpToDate. https://www.uptodate.com/contents/overview-of-medical-care-in-adults-with-diabetes-mellitus?search=diabetes&source=search_result&selectedTitle=1~150&usage_type=default&display_rank=1. Accessed December 2, 2018.

5. Horton WB, Subauste JS. Care of the athlete with type 1 diabetes mellitus: a clinical review. *Int J Endocrinol Metab.* 2016;14(2). doi:10.5812/ijem.36091.

6. Jimenez, CC, Corcoran MH, Crawley JT, et al. National Athletic Trainers' Association position statement: management of the athlete with type 1 diabetes mellitus. *J Athl Train.* 2007;42(4):536-545.

7. Lupsa BC, Inzucchi SE. Diabetic ketoacidosis and hyperosmolar hyperglycemic syndrome. *Endocr Emerg.* 2013:15-31. doi:10.1007/978-1-62703-697-9_2.

8. Colberg SR, Sigal RJ, Fernhall B, et al. Exercise and type 2 diabetes: the American College of Sports Medicine and the American Diabetes Association: joint position statement. *Diabetes Care.* 2010;33(12):e147-167.

6

Respiratory Emergencies

Francis Feld, DNP, CRNA, LAT, ATC, NRP

Chapter Key Words

- Asthma
- Hemothorax
- Pneumothorax
- Tension pneumothorax

Chapter Scenario

During a professional football game, the starting running back presents to the athletic trainer complaining of wheezing and difficulty breathing. The athlete has a known history of asthma, and the team physician is immediately summoned to evaluate him. The physician confirms an acute exacerbation of asthma, and the athlete is assisted from the field to an area out of public view. Paramedics assigned to the team sideline follow the medical staff and provide an albuterol nebulizer and supplemental oxygen. After 2 albuterol treatments, the athlete feels better and wants to return to the game. The team physician performs a quick physical examination and clears the athlete to return to competition. He completes the game without incident and performs well.

Scenario Resolution

This athlete had a known history of asthma, and the team medical staff was prepared to deal with an acute attack. Return to competition after treatment was indicated considering the sport level, and the team physician was also the treating physician, so he was aware of the athlete's medical condition. This may not be the case at other sport levels, so return-to-play decisions must be made at the local level, and caution is always advised.

Introduction

Air hunger seen with difficult breathing is a terrifying experience for both the patient and the health care professional providing care. Patients who are hypoxic can be combative and difficult to treat and control. Early recognition and management are necessary to prevent a manageable condition from deteriorating into a catastrophic event. Respiratory emergency conditions seen in athletics are either medical- or trauma-related.

The most common medical condition in this population is asthma, whereas blunt force trauma to the thorax can result in pleural injuries. Penetrating trauma to the thorax will usually result in pleural injury, but this type of trauma is rarely seen in athletics. This chapter will briefly examine airway management and recognition, and treatment of medical- and trauma-related respiratory emergencies. Airway management is a technique that requires

Feld F., Corso KM, Blanc RO
Non-Orthopedic Emergency Care in Athletics (pp 43-47).
© 2020 Taylor & Francis Group.

comprehensive education, and health care professionals working in the athletic arena should avail themselves of additional training in this vital area.

Airway Management

A patient who is conversing normally is said to have a *patent* airway. Patency refers to the patient's ability to breathe without obstruction. A patient may experience difficulty breathing and still have a patent airway. Signs of obstruction are snoring, sternal retractions, intercostal retractions, accessory muscle contractions, nasal flaring, and gurgling sounds. Snoring in the unconscious patient is caused by an upper airway obstruction and is managed in the short-term by either a chin lift or jaw thrust maneuver. The jaw thrust is stimulating and may arouse the unconscious patient. Gurgling indicates fluid in the upper airway and is managed by suctioning out the material. Other obstruction signs indicate a more complex pathology and are managed by treating the underlying condition.

Cyanosis, a bluish coloration of the skin and mucous membranes, is an ominous sign of hypoxia. It is a late sign and mandates definitive interventions to improve oxygenation and ventilation. Pulse oximetry is a low-cost, noninvasive monitor that is routinely used to assess the oxygen status of patients and should be readily available in the athletic arena. The *pulse oximeter* is a clip applied to a finger, and it measures the difference between saturated and desaturated hemoglobin by passing infrared and red light through the finger. Saturated hemoglobin absorbs infrared light at 990 nanometers, whereas desaturated hemoglobin absorbs red light at 660 nanometers. The gradient is an indication of saturated hemoglobin and is expressed as a percentage. Normal ranges for a healthy non-smoker are between 99% and 100%. Values lower than 94% should be treated with supplemental oxygen. Pulse oximetry assumes that the hemoglobin is saturated with oxygen, but other compounds, such as carbon monoxide, will bind to hemoglobin preferentially over oxygen and give false-positive readings.

Although pulse oximetry is a measure of oxygenation, ventilation is measured by carbon dioxide (CO_2) exchange at the alveolar level. Capnography monitors end tidal CO_2 with a nasal cannula. Normal CO_2 levels are 35 to 45 mm of mercury as measured by arterial blood gases, while end tidal CO_2 runs slightly lower due to normal physiological dead space. Capnography is expensive, and although normally found in most ambulances in the United States, it is not readily available in the athletic arena. Effective airway management results in a patient who has saturated hemoglobin and is ventilated. This can be accomplished in many ways and is crucial for optimal patient management.

Supplemental Oxygen Administration

The availability of supplemental oxygen at sporting events depends on many factors; although optimal, it is not mandatory. Oxygen tanks require proper storage and management and failure to do so can be dangerous. Oxygen tanks come in different sizes and those most commonly used outside the hospital are E and D tanks. Each tank has a regulator that reduces the tank pressure to a manageable level and a flow meter that supplies the oxygen device used. Tanks must be stored in proper holders and not subjected to extremes of temperature. If the regulator is damaged, the tank can become a deadly missile. Although oxygen is not flammable, it does support combustion, so no open flames or ignition sources should be in close proximity. Clearly labeled signage is required to indicate oxygen is in use. State practice laws may restrict the use of oxygen, so health care professionals must consider all these factors when deciding whether to use supplemental oxygen.

Oxygen tanks are made of aluminum and painted green. A full tank is pressurized to 2000 psi. The D tank holds approximately 360 L of oxygen, whereas the E tank holds approximately 625 L. The size of the D tank makes it convenient for sideline equipment bags, but its utility is suspect because it may be exhausted prior to emergency medical services (EMS) arrival. To estimate how long a D tank will last, multiply the pressure shown on the regulator by 0.2, and then divide by the flow rate. To estimate how long an E tank will last, multiply the pressure shown on the regulator by 0.3, and then divide by the flow rate. Although these are estimates, a full E tank will last twice as long as a full D tank.

Oxygen delivery devices include nasal cannulas, simple facemasks, reservoir facemasks, bag-valve masks (BVMs), supraglottic airways (SGA), and endotracheal tubes. The amount of oxygen delivered to the patient by each device is called the fraction of inspired oxygen (FiO_2) and varies with liter flow and device used. A nasal cannula is oxygen tubing with prongs that fit into the nares, with tubing loops that go around the ears. A simple facemask has vents for expiration and fits over the mouth and nose with an elastic strap that can be tightened for a snug seal around the head. A plastic bag attached to the reservoir facemask fills with oxygen and allows for a higher FiO_2 delivery. This mask also has vents for expiration. The reservoir bag does not have to fill completely for oxygen delivery.

All these devices allow a certain amount of rebreathing of CO_2 that prevents them from delivering an FiO_2 of 100%. A type of reservoir facemask that has valves over the vents is called a non-rebreathing facemask and will deliver up to 90% oxygen, but these are rarely used. Oxygen delivered through a secure airway, such as an SGA or endotracheal tubes with a BVM, will provide the highest FiO_2 possible. The BVM may be used with a facemask and an airway adjunct to ventilate a patient prior to the insertion of an SGA or endotracheal tube. Prior to using any of these tools, all health care professionals must review state practice acts. Endotracheal intubation and SGA insertion are advanced life support skills and are restricted to select health professionals in all states. Table 6-1 shows the flow rates and FiO$_2$ of each device.

Airway Adjuncts

Although a chin lift or jaw thrust maneuver will often relieve an airway obstruction, these are considered short-term measures, and both require an airway adjunct such as a nasopharyngeal airway (NPA) or oropharyngeal airway (OPA) for definitive management.

The NPA is a soft tube that is lubricated with a water-soluble gel and inserted along the most inferior aspect of the nares, which is the largest passageway. The bevel at the end of the NPA orients toward the septum and is usually inserted into the right nostril. If significant resistance is met upon insertion, the NPA should be withdrawn and inserted into the left nostril. Aligning the bevel with the septum requires rotating the NPA 180 degrees upon insertion, and after approximately half of the airway is inserted, the NPA is rotated into its original alignment and inserted until the flared end is flush with the nares. The diameter of the NPA should approximate the diameter of the patient's fifth finger, and the length is the distance from the nares to the earlobe. If an NPA is inserted forcefully or without adequate lubrication, a severe nosebleed may result. This bleeding will complicate airway management and must be avoided at all costs.

The OPA is inserted into the mouth over the tongue into the posterior oropharynx. Insertion may be aided with the use of a tongue depressor to retract the tongue upon insertion. Care must be taken to prevent injury to the hard palate of the upper mouth, especially in children. An intact gag reflex is an absolute contraindication for the use of the OPA. The length of the OPA is the distance from the corner of the mouth to the earlobe. An Internet search will easily provide pictures of both devices in place.

Sizes for both the NPA and the OPA are variable based on the manufacturer. The NPA may be 26 to 34 French (8.6-11.3 mm), or it may be small, medium, and large. The NPA is made of silicone and is non-latex. The OPA size may be 60 to 100 mm, or it could be small, medium, and large. The OPA is made of plastic.

Use of both airway adjunct types requires additional education and frequent review. The use of the BVM for mask ventilation is a difficult psychomotor skill to master and requires frequent review and practice.

Medical Respiratory Emergencies

Asthma is a common respiratory condition found in 1 of 13 adults and 1 of 12 children.[1] Triggers such as dust, pollen, chemicals, cold weather, and smoke cause asthma attacks. These triggers cause inflammation and swelling

TABLE 6-1. FLOW RATES AND FiO$_2$

DEVICE	FLOW RATE (L/M)	FiO$_2$ (%)
Nasal cannula	1-6	25-40
Simple facemask	6-10	40-60
Reservoir facemask	10-15	60-90
BVM with mask	10-15	80-100
BVM with SGA/ETT	10-15	100

Abbreviations: BVM, bag-valve mask; ETT, endotracheal tube; SGA, supragiottic airway.

that constrict the bronchial airways. Symptoms include wheezing, coughing, and difficulty breathing. Wheezing is noted when auscultating breath sounds with a stethoscope and may be in one or multiple lung fields. Wheezing that is audible without a stethoscope may indicate a more severe attack. Acute asthma attacks can be fatal, and 10 people in the United States die every day from asthma.[1] There is no cure for asthma, but with proper medication and monitoring, people with asthma can participate in any activity.

Medications are available for asthma management, and the treating physician will determine which combination is best for each patient. Short-acting beta agonist medications such as albuterol or Atrovent (ipratropium bromide) are called rescue inhalers and are used for the immediate management of an acute attack. These medications relax bronchial constriction and provide immediate relief. Asthmatics should have their rescue inhalers with them at all times. Health care professionals may keep the inhalers on the sidelines during practice or competition and assist the athlete with using the inhalers during an attack.

Maintenance medications include inhaled corticosteroids and long-acting beta agonists. Long-acting beta agonists are never administered without an inhaled corticosteroid; a commonly used example is fluticasone propionate and salmeterol inhaler. The corticosteroids control bronchial inflammation, whereas the long-term beta agonists prevent constriction. These medications may lead to a fungal infection in the mouth called *thrush*, and it is recommended that patients rinse their mouths with water after use. Despite proper long-term control, triggers may overwhelm the medication and cause an attack.

Management of an acute asthma attack includes administration of supplemental oxygen if available and assisting the athlete with the use of his or her rescue inhaler. Activating EMS is indicated if the symptoms are not immediately relieved with the rescue inhaler. EMS may administer albuterol, Atrovent, or a combination of both via nebulizer with supplemental oxygen. Transport to hospital

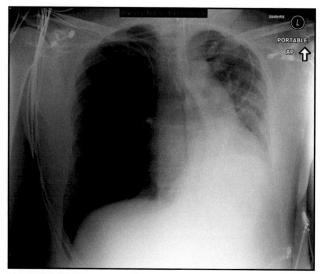

Figure 6-1. Tension pneumothorax.

is not necessary if symptoms are relieved completely, and the athlete should follow up with his or her physician for supplemental management. Acute asthma attacks often require oral corticosteroids and antibiotics. Return to competition after an attack is problematic and should be undertaken with caution.

Traumatic Respiratory Emergencies

Blunt force trauma to the chest can result in a pneumothorax. Injury to the lung can cause air to enter the potential space between the pleural membrane and the lung. This air expands the space and results in what is commonly called a collapsed lung. Although a rib fracture may be associated with a pneumothorax, it is not an absolute finding. Symptoms of a pneumothorax include difficulty breathing, pain that worsens on deep inspiration, pain radiating to the back or shoulder, and coughing. Absent or reduced breath sounds on stethoscope auscultation over the injured area are diagnostic. Stethoscope auscultation in the athletic environment may be difficult secondary to ambient noise, so this procedure should occur in a private area of the venue.

Diagnosis is confirmed at a hospital with a chest X-ray and may require placement of a chest tube. Chest tube placement depends on the size of the pneumothorax, symptoms, and patient status. Small-bore chest tubes are favored over large-bore tubes and contribute to improved patient comfort and shorter hospital stays.[2] A thoracic surgeon should evaluate any patient sustaining a pneumothorax as soon as possible.

A spontaneous simple pneumothorax may occur without trauma. This condition is usually found in young, tall, thin males, and the only complaint is difficulty breathing. The patient will report a sudden onset and deny injury. Smoking and drug use may be comorbidities. After initial

treatment, the condition can reoccur, and a thoracic surgeon my elect surgical interventions to prevent recurrence.

If blood enters the pleural space, a hemothorax can result. Symptoms are the same as a pneumothorax, and differentiation in the field is difficult. Percussion of the chest may produce a tympanic sound in the simple pneumothorax, whereas a hemothorax would produce a dull sound. As with stethoscope auscultation, percussion requires a quiet environment and is subjective. A hemothorax requires a large-bore chest tube, as the small-bore tubes will clot off easily with blood.

A simple pneumothorax and a hemothorax may progress into a life-threatening tension pneumothorax (Figure 6-1). The air or blood in the pleural space expands to the level of occluding the great vessels of the chest, including the aorta. This can lead to circulatory collapse and death. Symptoms include pain, severe difficulty breathing, tachycardia, tachypnea, hypotension, absent breath sounds, and altered levels of consciousness. A very late sign is the trachea deviated away from the affected side.

Immediate treatment requires needle decompression of the tension pneumothorax. A 14-gauge intravenous catheter is inserted into the second intercostal space in the midaxillary line until the pleural space is entered. A sudden release of pressure indicates proper placement of the catheter and is heard audibly. The stylet is removed from the intravenous catheter, and a one-way valve or stopcock is attached. When the pressure is relieved, the valve or stopcock is closed to prevent reentry of air through the catheter. If pressure increases again, the valve or stopcock is reopened to allow pressure release. Recently, a catheter with a built-in ball valve has been marketed and may prove superior to the long, 14-gauge intravenous technique.

Needle decompression of the tension pneumothorax requires specialized education, and health care professionals should consult their state practice acts. This technique is within the paramedic scope of practice.

CHAPTER SUMMARY

Respiratory emergencies may be life-threatening and are not rare. Health care professionals working athletic events must be aware of the health history of all team members and prepare to treat any acute events that may arise. The inability to breathe is terrifying for the patient, and the treating professional must remain calm and act definitively. Early activation of EMS is always indicated. Many of the techniques and equipment described in this chapter may be beyond the scope of practice for many, but familiarization with the basics is mandatory for all.

CHAPTER REVIEW QUESTIONS

1. In which nostril is an NPA usually inserted?
2. What is the difference in FiO_2 delivered by a nasal cannula and a simple facemask?
3. In a pneumothorax, _____ enters the pleural space, whereas in a hemothorax, _____ enters the pleural space.
4. Albuterol is considered a _____ inhaler.
5. What major symptom differentiates a tension pneumothorax from a simple pneumothorax?

ANSWERS

1. Right
2. 25% to 40% vs 40% to 60%
3. Air and blood
4. Rescue
5. Cardiovascular collapse

REFERENCES

1. Asthma and Allergy Foundation of America. https://www.aafa.org. Accessed August 2018.
2. MacDuff A, Arnold A, Harvey J; BTS Pleural Disease Guideline Group. Management of spontaneous pneumothorax: British Thoracic Society pleural disease guideline 2010. *Thorax.* 2010;65(suppl 2):ii8-31.

7

Environmental Conditions

Aaron V. Mares, MD and Shane Hennessy, DO

CHAPTER KEY WORDS

- Altitude
- Cold
- Environmental
- Heat
- Lightning

CHAPTER SCENARIO

A 17-year-old male high school football player becomes dizzy and lightheaded, and starts vomiting during practice. On initial evaluation, he appears to be confused and cannot stand up without leaning on a teammate.

SCENARIO RESOLUTION

Possible heat illness is immediately recognized. The athlete is moved to a shaded area, and his equipment is removed. Vital signs show a slight tachycardia of 110 beats/minute, blood pressure of 118/68, and a rectal temperature of 105°F. Ice bath immersion is completed, and his core temperature drops to 102°F within 9 minutes. After cooling, he is transported to the nearest local hospital via ambulance for further monitoring.

INTRODUCTION

Medical professionals share a unique objective when caring for the athlete. Although the competitor's focus is sharply aimed at winning, the medical professional is concentrating on success *and* safety. Many factors can alter the athlete's success, health, and safety while competing. Outcomes on the field of play are directly related to factors that include conditioning, strength, ability, and preparation. Much less considered is the effect the environment has on health, safety, and performance.

Environmental conditions not only affect how an athlete performs, but may also put an athlete at significant risk for a catastrophic medical complication. Heat illness, hypothermia, altitude sickness, and lightning are some of the more common conditions experienced, and many other environmental risk factors affect the athlete population. In this chapter, we will discuss temperature extremes, high altitude, and lightning, with goal of providing a basic understanding and systematic approach to their management.

Exertional Heat Illness

Exertional heat illness (EHI) is a common environmental-related condition with which all medical providers need to be familiar. Although debated and not universally agreed upon, EHI is often thought of as a continuum. Regardless, degrees of severity vary from mild to moderate to severe.[1,2]

Feld F., Gorse KM, Blanc RO
Non-Orthopedic Emergency Care in Athletics (pp 49-54).
© 2020 Taylor & Francis Group.

TABLE 7-1. TEMPERATURE ACTION PROTOCOL

WBGT	RECOMMENDED ACTION
65°F to 72°F	Monitor high-risk individuals
72°F to 78°F	General risk rises for all competitors
78°F to 82°F	Remove high-risk athletes from competition
82°F to 86°F	Remove unacclimated, unfit competitors
86°F to 90°F	Limit fit, acclimated competitors
> 90°F	Stop all activities

Abbreviation: WBGT, wet-bulb globe temperature.
Adapted from Armstrong L, Casa DJ, Milliard-Stafford M, Moran D, Pyne S, Roberts W. American College of Sports Medicine position stand. Exertional heat illness during training and competition. *Med Sci Sport Exerc.* 2007;39(3):556-572.

Heat cramps and heat rash are forms of mild EHI. Heat cramps are common, but do not predispose the athlete to more severe forms of EHI. These painful, involuntary skeletal muscle contractions are typically brought on by prolonged exertion and more commonly occur at higher temperatures. Heat cramps are treated with rest, rehydration, stretching, and massage. The athlete may return to play when properly rehydrated and the cramping has subsided.[3]

Heat rash is simply a pruritic, maculopapular, erythematous rash that develops in areas of maximal warmth and tight-fitting clothing. The sweat glands become clogged, swell, and rupture. This self-limiting rash is best treated with loose fitting clothing and antihistamines.[2,4]

The clinical signs and symptoms of moderate and severe EHI (heat exhaustion and heat stroke) often overlap. Athletes commonly present with some combination of profuse sweating, lethargy, headache, dizziness, cool and clammy skin, nausea, tachycardia, hypotension, hyperventilation, and an elevated core body temperature (CBT). These are the signs of the vascular strain the body is experiencing in an attempt to thermoregulate.

Ominous signs of potential progression toward heat stroke include cessation of profuse sweating and the lack of spontaneous cooling when exertion has been stopped.[1,2,4] The American College of Sports Medicine (ACSM) defines heat stroke as an elevated core body temperature greater than 40°C, or 104°F, plus central nervous system alterations such as seizure or disordered thought. Early recognition of EHI is crucial in successful treatment and prevention of long-term effects or death. The suspicion of EHI for any collapsed athlete should be high, and early CBT measurement is needed. Rectal temperatures are considered the gold standard measurement of CBT, and treatment must be provided rapidly when the suspicion or diagnosis is made.

Thermoregulation occurs through radiation, conduction, convection, and evaporation, with the latter 3 employed in the medical professional's cooling efforts. In evaporation, the most commonly understood form, heat is lost as liquid changes phase to vapor, such as during sweating. Conduction is the transfer of heat between unmoving objects. This can be achieved by cold-water immersion, ice vests, or simply ice packs within the groin and axilla. Convection is the transfer of heat from an object to moving air or water. This is classically accomplished with the use of a cooling fan, mist, or even immersion within a cold river or creek.

Early treatment, ideally within less than 30 minutes, has profound effects on return to normal thermoregulation and prevention of progression to heat stroke. The gold standard of treatment is cooling performed by full-body ice water immersion. The athlete should be removed from activity and taken to a shaded area if possible. If ice-water immersion is not available, other forms of cooling, such as misting, fanning, and ice packs, should be undertaken. Attempts to cool continue until the CBT reaches 39°C, or 102.2°F, and then the athlete may be transferred. It is important to avoid antipyretics, as this condition is a result of the overproduction of heat, and the body's hypothalamic set point is unaffected, rendering medications such as acetaminophen more detrimental than beneficial.

Rehydration is another important step in treatment of exertional heat illness. A rehydration goal of 1 to 2 L/hour is recommended. This fluid should contain 20 to 30 mEq/L of sodium, 2 to 5 mEq/L of potassium, and 5% to 10% carbohydrate. Most commercially sold sports drink fit these criteria.[3]

Athletes who are diagnosed and respond to treatment of exertional heat illness should avoid further exertion for the next 24 to 48 hours to avoid the increased, albeit transient, risk of recurrent EHI.[1]

Activity planning and reduction should be guided by the wet-bulb globe temperature (WBGT). The frequency of EHI increases proportionally with the increase in WBGT, which is calculated with the following formula[5]:

$$\text{WBGT} = (\text{wet bulb temp} \times 0.7) + (\text{dry bulb} \times 0.1) + (\text{black bulb} \times 0.2)$$

The WBGT represents humidity, dry bulb is air temperature, and black bulb is radiant heat. High-risk individuals include obese athletes, those with poor physical fitness or a recent episode of heat illness, athletes with a concomitant febrile illness, and those taking medications or supplements that alter thermoregulation, such as antihistamines, caffeine, and diuretics. It is generally considered low risk for heat illness when the WBGT is less than 65°F, but the ACSM offers the following recommendations for temperatures above this threshold (Table 7-1).[1]

Finally, other preventative steps may be taken to reduce the risk of EHI in athletes. A period of acclimatization of at least 4 to 5 days is recommended; however, 10 to 14 days is closer to ideal. The ACSM has recommended proper hydration of 16-oz water or sports beverage several hours before exercise, plus 13 to 27 oz/hour during activity.

Hypothermia

Activity in cold temperatures places athletes at risk of hypothermia or other peripheral cold injuries. Unfortunately, our physiologic response to low temperature is less effective when compared to our warm-weather adaptive changes. Luckily, the incidence of cold injury is low in athletics, with hypothermia and frostbite accounting for only 20% of cross-country skiing injuries and fewer than 5% of injuries in mountaineers.[6] Other at-risk events include ultramarathons and triathlons, particularly due to the duration of competition and swimming. With the increasing popularity of these activities, there should continue to be heightened awareness of the physiologic changes our bodies go through in cold temperatures, as well as the classic injuries.

Our bodies transfer heat in 4 primary ways. In the setting of cold injury, we primarily focus on convective heat loss. Tolerance to cold varies by the individual and hinges on duration of exposure, environmental factors, and preexisting risk factors unique to the athlete. The amount of heat exchanged from our skin to the environment is directly affected by the ambient temperature, humidity, wind speed, precipitation, and the insulating properties of our clothing.[6,7] The human body works to maintain a CBT near 37°C, or 98.6°F. To combat a dropping core temperature, our bodies must create more heat and decrease lost heat. To increase heat production, the body involuntarily begins to shiver. We can additionally increase heat production by exertion. To minimize heat loss, peripheral vessel vasoconstriction occurs when the skin temperatures reach 35°C or below to shunt blood away from the skin and subcutaneous tissue. The most challenging environment combines cold, wind, and wet. Temperature alone cannot be the only factor considered, and a perfect example is *wind chill*, the actual temperature when wind is factored. It is calculated by the following formula:

$$WC\ (°F) = 35.74 + 0.6215T - 35.75(V^{0.16}) + 0.4275T(V^{0.16})$$

where T is air temperature and V is the wind speed (mph).

Other risk factors for cold injury include inactivity, inappropriate attire, impaired thermoregulation, previous cold injury, age, and preexisting medical conditions. Athletes with prior frostbite have a 2- to 4-fold increased risk of repeat injury. Young children and adults older than 60 years have a greater risk. Our shiver response can be blunted by hypoglycemia, poor caloric intake, and endocrine abnormalities, leading to poor heat production.

Disorders such as hyperhidrosis, chronic dermatologic conditions, and low-percent body fat may lead to increased heat loss. Athletes with known reactive airway disease have an increased risk of cold-induced bronchospasm. Finally, there is an increased rate of cardiovascular events secondary to cold-induced increases in mean arterial pressure, total peripheral resistance, and increased cardiac output and oxygen demand.[8]

Hypothermia is defined as a drop in CBT below 35°C. In the early stages, shivering, lethargy, apathy, and cold extremities can occur.[9] However, as this progresses, the athlete experiences confusion, impaired gross motor control, and slurred speech. Core temperatures below 35°C lead to bradycardia, hypotension, and decreased cardiac output, which strain the myocardium and predispose the patient to spontaneous dysrhythmias. In the severe stages, hypothermia causes pulmonary edema, muscle rigidity, and loss of consciousness. General considerations in immediate management include ABCs (Airway, Breathing, Circulation), gentle handling of affected extremities, and removal of any wet clothing.[6,9]

Rewarming is either passive or active, depending on the degree of hypothermia. Passive external rewarming is for athletes with a CBT of greater than 32°C, and consists of removing wet clothing and covering the victim with warm blankets. The goal rewarming rate is 0.5°C to 2.0°C/hour. Active external rewarming consists of fires, hot water bottles, and heating pads. Active core rewarming is accomplished in a controlled setting with intravenous 5% dextrose in normal saline warmed to 40°C to 42°C, inhalation of warmed oxygen, or, more intensively, a warmed peritoneal lavage. These active forms of rewarming are reserved for CBTs below 32°C.

Care must be taken to avoid *afterdrop*, a phenomenon that occurs with active external rewarming. In chronic hypothermia, dehydration leads to general hypotension and hypovolemia. The cold extremity vessels are vasoconstricted, and the blood returning is cold and acidic. By rewarming the extremity, there is peripheral vasodilation and a resultant drop in CBT, pH, and blood pressure, which decrease coronary perfusion and increase risk of arrhythmia. For this reason, it is imperative to rewarm the core first before addressing the extremities.[9]

Peripheral cold injuries can be further broken down into freezing and nonfreezing injuries. Some nonfreezing injuries (often termed *cold–wet injuries*) such as trench foot are not high yield in athletics, as these tend to occur after more than 12 hours of exposure. Other nonfreezing injuries include chilblains and cold urticaria.[6,10] Chilblains are superficial, cold-induced erythrocyanotic skin lesions that develop within 24 hours of cold exposure. Athletes experience tender, pruritic erythematous papules in sites of cold exposure. There is concern that blistering and ulceration may develop secondary infection; however, the condition is otherwise self-limiting. Athletes should avoid further cold exposure, and lesions resolve within 2 to 3 weeks. Cold urticaria, much like chilblains, develops on exposed skin and presents as erythematous, pruritic hives. However, these typically develop within minutes of exposure. These are also self-limiting, and treatment consists of removing from cold, limiting reexposure, and giving antihistamines for pruritus.[10]

Frostbite, generally considered the most common cold injury, falls into the freezing category of peripheral cold injuries. Frostbite develops when the skin and deeper tissue reach temperatures at or below 0°C, or 31°F.[6] The most commonly affected areas include ears, nose, cheeks, chin, fingers, and toes. Athletes will initially complain of numbness, cold, insensate skin with difficulty moving digits, and white or gray discoloration of surrounding skin. It is further classified into the following 4 stages:

- First-degree injuries are limited to the epidermis.
- Second-degree injury is characterized by full-thickness involvement of the dermis, leading to edema and the formation of clear blisters. Over a 2- to 3-week period, these blisters contract and form dark eschars. Sequelae include persistent cold sensitivity, paresthesia, and hyperhidrosis.
- Third-degree frostbite is distinguished from second degree by formation of hemorrhagic blisters, deep burning pain on rewarming, and thick gangrenous eschar formation.
- Fourth-degree frostbite involves deeper muscle, bone, and tendons.

Prehospital management consists of removing the athlete from cold environment and removing any wet clothing. Handle the affected area with care, as vigorous manipulation of involved tissue will lead to further damage. Do not begin rewarming until there is no further risk of cold exposure, and be careful with active rewarming, as the skin is insensate and will burn without the athlete knowing. When in a controlled setting, the affected skin may be actively rewarmed with warm water immersion at a temperature around 98°F. Too-high temperatures may risk burning, lead to increased pain, and will not hasten the process. Tetanus prophylaxis is recommended, but antibiotics remain controversial. Further wound management should be handled by an expert.[7,10]

High-Altitude Illness

Competitive and recreational athletes exerting at elevation face certain risks to health and performance. Health care personnel should be familiar with common altitude-related illnesses such as acute mountain sickness, high-altitude cerebral edema, and high-altitude pulmonary edema, as well as the physiologic effects of elevation, risk factors, and preventative measures of such conditions.

At high altitudes, our bodies are exposed to lower levels of ambient oxygen and increased thermal radiation. The primary driving force behind high-altitude illness (HAI) is believed to be hypoxemia, secondary to low partial pressure of inspired oxygen, which acts as the driving force behind oxygen diffusion as we inhale. As elevation increases, the barometric pressure and available oxygen fall.[11] During activity, tissue oxygen demands are high. At high altitude, the marked reduction in pressure and oxygen availability results in tissue hypoxia. An individual's response to high altitude is highly variable and depends on individual fitness levels, exertion on arrival at altitude, prior residence at low altitude, sensitivity to hypoxia, the blood's oxygen-carrying capacity, nutritional status, obesity, and prior episodes of HAI.[11-13]

The most important preventative measure is slow ascent, especially at altitudes greater than 2000 to 3000 m. Consensus guidelines recommend an ascent of 300 to 600 m/day when above 3000 m. In addition, for every 1000 m gained, there should be a planned 24 hours of rest. Maintaining appropriate hydration is imperative at high elevation, as there is an increase of insensible losses and thus an increased risk of dehydration. Appropriate clothing and application of sunscreen reduce the risk of sun-related injuries, which have high incidence due to increased ultraviolet radiation at high elevation. Finally, and typically reserved for those with prior cases of HAI or a need to ascend rapidly, medications (eg, acetazolamide, dexamethasone, and nifedipine) have been used to decrease the incidence of HAI. Special consideration must be taken with use of acetazolamide and dexamethasone, as these substances are banned by the World Anti-Doping Agency.[13]

Acute mountain sickness (AMS) is the most common form of HAI and is considered the early, more benign side of a spectrum containing high-altitude cerebral edema (HACE). AMS is characterized by a high-altitude headache plus one of the following: nausea or vomiting, fatigue, dizziness, or insomnia. Generally, this is a delayed reaction occurring 6 to 12 hours after arrival; however, it may present as quickly as 1 to 2 hours or as late as 24 hours. AMS is self-limiting, and, if no further ascent is obtained, the symptoms will gradually resolve within 48 hours.[11,13] This is not considered life-threatening, but it may significantly impact performance. Aside from resting, symptomatic treatment is provided for issues such as headaches and nausea. Concern for HACE arises if the athlete develops ataxia, altered level of consciousness, or other signs of neurologic impact. These symptoms develop as a result of brain edema secondary to increased permeability of the blood–brain barrier. The mechanism of the increased permeability is not completely understood.[13] This is considered a medical emergency, and early recognition is critical. The definitive treatment of HACE is descent; however, this is not always possible, given level of consciousness and weather. If not possible, supplemental oxygen or hyperbaric therapy may be applied. In addition, dexamethasone may be initiated until descent is completed.[11,13]

High-altitude pulmonary edema is the abnormal accumulation of fluid in the lungs secondary to a breakdown in the pulmonary blood–gas barrier.[11] This is separate from the AMS-HACE continuum and is believed to be secondary to maladaptive responses to hypobaric hypoxia experienced in high altitude. High-altitude pulmonary edema generally develops 2 to 5 days after arrival and is characterized by shortness of breath, cough, and poor exercise tolerance.[14] Like HACE, high-altitude pulmonary edema is a medical emergency and can rapidly progress to severe shortness of breath at rest. Additional signs are tachycardia, tachypnea, and a low-grade fever. First-line treatment is rest and oxygen. Again, definitive treatment is descent, but hyperbaric therapy is an option if oxygen is not available and descent is delayed. Finally, nifedipine may be used; however, the clinical evidence is modest, and, in most cases, does not offer benefit compared with oxygen and descent.[13,14]

Lightning

Mother Nature can be most unpredictable regarding severe-weather storms. Lightning strikes can lead to both injuries and death. Approximately 15% of all lightning deaths occur during sporting events. This is concerning, as many of these fatalities could be avoided if proper precautions were taken. In 2013, the National Athletic Trainers' Association released a position statement outlining lightning safety recommendations. They included the following guidelines:

1. Establish a lightning-specific emergency action plan for each venue.
2. Ensure lightning and general weather awareness.
3. Prepare large-venue planning protocol.
4. Provide first aid.

Currently, we have access to weather forecast resources at our fingertips. However, a team or individual may be traveling to a remote location, and proper steps need to be taken to ensure safety. During a lightning storm, take shelter indoors, such as in an enclosed building, vehicle, or even a basement. If those are not readily available, alternatives may include picnic shelters or even covered bus stops.

If a lightning strike is visualized or thunder is heard, activity should be halted for a minimum of 30 minutes. The clock starts after the most recent event. An individual should be put in charge of coordinating the evacuation of a venue. These protocols should be made, reviewed, and practiced prior to holding an event.

Should lightning strike an individual, a first responder needs to make sure his or her safety is not compromised before attending to a victim. When it is determined as safe, the victim should be moved to a safe location. An automated external defibrillator should be available, and basic life support should be initiated if indicated.

Chapter Summary

Environmental conditions play a large role in the management of the athlete. A medical professional must be aware of the clear and present dangers to which an athlete may be exposed and how to appropriately manage these individuals. Be aware of local and forecasted weather conditions, and, if traveling to an unfamiliar environment, research and gain a better understanding of the conditions with which you and the athlete may be confronted.

Chapter Review Questions

1. What is the gold standard for taking an individual's body temperature if heat illness is suspected?
2. The American College of Sports Medicine defines heat stroke as a temperature greater than 40°C (104°F) plus what?
3. True or False: In hypothermia, it is imperative to warm the core first before addressing the extremities.
4. What is the definitive treatment for high-altitude cerebral edema?
5. An athletic event should be suspended for how many minutes from the last witnessed lightning strike or sound of thunder?

Answers

1. Rectal temperature
2. Central nervous system alteration
3. True
4. Descent
5. 30 minutes

References

1. Armstrong L, Casa DJ, Milliard-Stafford M, Moran D, Pyne S, Roberts W. American College of Sports Medicine position stand. Exertional heat illness during training and competition. *Med Sci Sport Exerc.* 2007;39(3):556-572.
2. Asplund CA, O'Connor FG, Noakes TD. Exercise-associated collapse: an evidence-based review and primer for clinicians. *Br J Sports Med.* 2011;45(14):1157-1162.
3. Schwellnus MP, Drew N, Collins M. Muscle cramping in athletes—risk factors, clinical assessment, and management. *Clin Sports Med.* 2008;27(1):183-194.
4. Casa DJ, DeMartini JK, Bergeron MF, et al. National Athletic Trainers' Association position statement: exertional heat illnesses. *J Athl Train.* 2015;50(9):986-1000.

5. Racinais S, Alonso JM, Coutts AJ, et al. Consensus recommendations on training and competing in the heat. *Br J Sports Med.* 2015;49(18):1164-1173.

6. Fudge MD, Bennett BL, Simanis JP, Roberts WO. Medical evaluation for exposure extremes:cold. *Clin J Sport Med.* 2015;25:432-436.

7. Castellani JW, Young AJ, Ducharme MB, et al. Position stand: prevention of cold injuries during exercise. *Med Sci Sports Exerc.* 2006;37:2012-2029.

8. Castellani JW, Young AJ. Health and performance challenges during sports training and competition in cold weather. *Br J Sports Med.* 2012;46:788-791.

9. Brown DJ, Brugger H, Boyd J, Paal P. Accidental hypothermia. *N Engl J Med.* 2012;367(20):1930-8.

10. Harirchi I, Arvin A, Vash JH, Zafarmand V. Frostbite: incidence and predisposing factors in mountaineers. *Br J Sports Med.* 2005;39:898-901.

11. Bartsch P, Swenson ER. Clinical practice: acute high-altitude illnesses. *N Engl J Med.* 2013;368:2294-2302.

12. West JB, American College of Physicians, American Physiological Society. The physiologic basis of high-altitude diseases. *Ann Intern Med.* 2004;141(10):789-800.

13. Koehle MS, Cheng I, Sporer B. Canadian academy of sport and exercise medicine position statement: athletes at high altitude. *Clin J Sport Med.* 2014;24(2):120-127.

14. Stream JO, Grissom CK. Update on high-altitude pulmonary edema: pathogenesis, prevention, and treatment. *Wilderness Environ Med.* 2008;19(4):293-303.

8

Shock

Timothy Rausch, MSN, CRNP

CHAPTER KEY WORDS

- Exercise-induced anaphylaxis
- Methicillin-resistant *Staphylococcus aureus*

CHAPTER SCENARIO

You are the athletic trainer for the Pine Hollow Fighting Bulldogs football team. The team is playing its archrival, the Sun Valley Raging Lions. The team is keyed up for this annual Saturday night event. The stands are filled on both sides, and the energy in the air can be palpated. It is a hot, humid night, and the team has been practicing all afternoon. By game time, the team has been at it for hours, with few breaks and little nourishment.

The game gets underway, and the players are energized. "Touchdown" Ted Turner, the star quarterback, is particularly hyped. With a good showing, his acceptance to State College is almost guaranteed. The game is going well for the Bulldogs, and Touchdown Ted is at the top of his game. Just prior to halftime, he is sacked on a failed third down conversion by a particularly hefty middle linebacker. As he is exiting the field, he collapses. Suddenly, you are the center of attention. The team and crowd look at you to react. What is your first response?

As you approach him, he is surrounded by his teammates yelling for you to do something. You notice that he is unresponsive. Primary assessment reveals that his airway is open, respirations are shallow and rapid, and his pulse is weak and rapid. His skin is cool and clammy. What is your diagnosis? What is your next action?

You turn him supine and elevate his legs. The ambulance crew comes out onto the field and administers oxygen. Vital signs show his pulse to be 140/min, respiratory rate is 40/min, and blood pressure is 70/palpation. They initiate intravenous fluid wide open. Secondary assessment reveals guarding when palpating his abdomen. Does this change your differential diagnosis? Does this change your treatment approach?

SCENARIO RESOLUTION

After 2 liters of intravenous fluids, he begins to respond. He complains of severe abdominal pain. Emergency medical services staff take him to the emergency department. They determine that his hemoglobin and hematocrit is low. He is taken for a computed tomography scan and is found to have a ruptured spleen. He is admitted for observation and potential surgery.

Discussion

Long, outdoor activity in a warm environment is suspicious for dehydration. This is heightened because the focus is on a rival game and not on fluid replacement. The quarterback is the star player, and his adrenalin is running high. After an hour or so playing in the warm, humid climate, he is likely dehydrated. However, during the last play, he

Feld F., Gorse KM, Blanc RO
Non-Orthopedic Emergency Care in Athletics (pp 55-63).
© 2020 Taylor & Francis Group.

is tackled by a hefty linebacker. This detail could easily be missed if the athletic trainer is not paying attention.

Regardless of the underlying etiology, this player is clearly in shock. The first-line treatment is the same. Maintain airway, breathing, and circulation. Placing him supine and elevating his feet assists in shunting blood from the periphery into the central circulation. Suspicion of cervical spine injury is low, as he was ambulating prior to collapse. It is clear that he requires fluid resuscitation; however, oral replacement is dangerous in a person with altered mental status because of the risk of aspiration. Therefore, intravenous fluid replacement is the preferred method of volume resuscitation. The key to making the correct diagnosis is in the history. Shock due to dehydration would be less likely to occur acutely. However, gathering history from the referee would add information to make the diagnosis clearer.

Other Considerations

Concussion/Closed Head Injury

Although this would explain the sudden loss of consciousness, it does not explain the hypotension or tachycardia.

Other Types of Shock

Septic shock would present with other prodromal symptoms such as fever and malaise prior to collapse. Neurogenic shock may present with sudden collapse; however, it would be accompanied by severe neurological symptoms such as paresthesia or paralysis. Cardiogenic shock would explain some of these symptoms but it would not explain the abdominal pain.

Anaphylaxis

This would explain the tachycardia and hypotension; however, it does not explain the sudden collapse and would be accompanied by wheezing, urticaria, or rash.

Shock

The textbook definition of shock is simply *inadequate tissue perfusion*; however, shock is a very complex syndrome. In its simplest terms, a state of shock arises when blood flow to vital tissues does not supply adequate nutrients, specifically glucose and oxygen, to the cells. Shock can be defined by the means of restriction, such as cardiogenic shock, which results from decreased cardiac output; hypovolemic shock, resulting from decreased circulatory volume leading to inadequate peripheral blood flow; neurogenic shock that results from vascular dilation and decreased systemic vascular resistance; and septic shock as a response to a pathogen, which causes vascular dilation, increased capillary permeability, and increased cellular metabolism. The result of these syndromes is nutritional and oxygen starvation of the body's cells. This sets off a cascade of

events that, if left unchecked, rapidly progresses to massive cellular death and the individual's eventual demise. Although shock can rapidly progress, intervention by the athletic trainer can halt the process. The key is early recognition and intervention, with an adequate recovery period.

Shock on the Cellular Level

Shock is a cascade of events that can lead to cellular death. To survive, cells require 3 essential components: oxygen, glucose, and water, as shown in the following formula:

$$C_6H_{12}O_6 + 6O_2 \rightarrow 6CO_2 + 6H_2O + Energy$$

In addition to receiving essential nutrients, cells must be able to excrete byproducts and waste. Normal, aerobic metabolism produces waste products such as CO_2; ATP, or energy; and sulfates. When the body is in a state of homeostasis, these products are carried away by the circulation and excreted mainly by the liver and kidneys. However, in a state of low blood flow, these wastes and byproducts accumulate in the cells and interstitial fluid, causing electrolyte disturbances, fluid shifts, and acidosis.

During anaerobic metabolism, ATP is generated at an accelerated rate. This inefficient use of resources produces lactate and causes the blood pH to fall. The resulting metabolic acidosis causes peripheral vasoconstriction, precapillary sphincter failure, increased capillary permeability, and peripheral pooling of blood. A drop in cellular pH also causes membrane dysfunction and sodium pump failure; therefore, extracellular potassium and intracellular sodium increase. With a higher intracellular sodium concentration, water is drawn into the cell by osmosis, causing intravascular dehydration and cellular edema. Cells begin to lyse, and intracellular enzymes leak into the extracellular fluid. These enzymes erode the capillary endothelium, worsening peripheral edema. This further depletes the intravascular volume, and the shock response cycle continues (Figure 8-1).

As the cascade escalates, oxygen use by the cells becomes increasingly tedious, further shifting to anaerobic metabolism and acidosis. The body activates neurohumoral, negative feedback mechanisms in an attempt to correct the hypotension. Decreased circulatory volume further limits the compromised flow of oxygen to the cells. In septic, anaphylactic, and neurogenic shocks, the resultant vasodilation exacerbates the already-depleted intravascular volume. Profound hypotension ensues, and vital organs begin to fail. The extreme shift in electrolytes inhibits the function of intracellular enzymes. Cells begin to lose their ability to absorb nutrients and rid themselves of waste. Moreover, capillary flow becomes sluggish due to increased permeability and increased vascular viscosity. This, in turn, activates the clotting cascade, resulting in disseminated intravascular coagulation, which not only clots many smaller vessels, but also depletes circulating clotting components, producing even more uncontrolled hemorrhage. Finally, the deluge of enzymes exiting the cells destroys

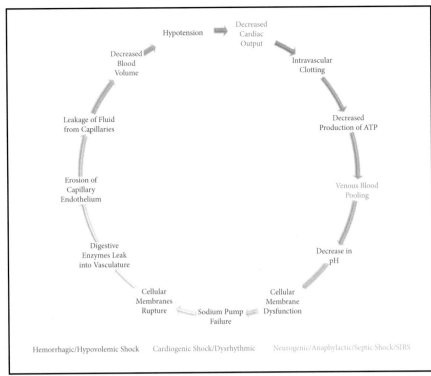

Figure 8-1. Biologic pathology of shock syndrome.

the cell membrane and the surrounding tissues. Anaerobic metabolism is used as a final effort for cellular survival but produces even more lactic acid and electrolyte shifts. The cycle continues until the environment becomes too hostile for the cells to survive. The victim becomes unconscious and, without rapid intervention, death is imminent.

Much as when cells are oxygen deprived, the inability to use glucose initiates a catastrophic set of events in cells. Glucose delivery is inhibited by the same mechanisms as oxygen delivery: low volume and low flow. Further, most tissues have limited, readily available glucose stores. Shock states, such as sepsis, increase cellular metabolism, thus exacerbating an already-broken system. When glucose stores are consumed, cells will revert to proteins, lipids, and other nontraditional sources for energy. Use of these is highly inefficient and produces toxic byproducts such as lactic acid, uric acid, and ammonia.

Classifications of Shock

Shock can be classified in a variety of ways; often, it is classified via etiology (Table 8-1). However, within any classification system, more than one shock state can exist simultaneously in the human body.

Hypovolemic Shock

Hypovolemic shock is one of the most frequent types of shock that an athletic trainer may encounter. Hypovolemic shock can be either hemorrhagic or non-hemorrhagic. Hemorrhagic, as the name implies, is the loss of whole blood. This is frequently the result of a traumatic insult, causing either external or internal bleeding. External hemorrhage results from lacerations, open fractures, or other types of external traumas that disrupt major vessels and create an external pathway for blood to escape. Internal hemorrhage is often due to blunt trauma. Detecting external hemorrhage is more subtle and more difficult. Unfortunately, internal injuries can be erroneously dismissed as bruises or contusions. Common sites of internal hemorrhage include solid organs, such as the pancreas and liver; large bones, such as the femur or pelvis; and hollow organs, such as lungs or bowel. When hemorrhagic events occur in sports, the quick recognition and treatment by the athletic trainer can turn a potential tragedy into a manageable event with a good outcome (Box 8-1).

Although hemorrhagic shock is frequently due to a loss of whole blood, it can also be the result of loss of plasma or other fluids. Burn injury can result in acute fluid loss. When a thermal burn occurs, the epidermis is disrupted, allowing massive loss of plasma externally. A similar example, not foreign to athletes, is dehydration, whereby fluid loss via the skin's sweating is not replenished.

In addition to blood volume loss resulting in a reduction in perfusion pressure, there is also a loss of oxygen-carrying capacity due to a loss of erythrocytes. As the body's defenses attempt to combat the hypovolemic state, fluid shifts from intracellular and interstitial spaces into the vasculature. Although this may partially or completely replace the lost blood volume, it does not replace the lost erythrocytes, and therefore does not restore the oxygen-carrying capacity. For example, individuals with coronary artery

TABLE 8-1. CLASSIFICATIONS OF SHOCK

ETIOLOGY	TYPE OF SHOCK
Hypovolemic	• Hemorrhagic • Non-hemorrhagic
Distributive	• Septic • Systemic inflammatory response syndrome (SIRS) • Anaphylactic • Neurogenic
Cardiogenic	• Cardiomyopathic • Dysrhythmic
Obstructive	• Pulmonary vascular • Mechanical

BOX 8-1. HEMORRHAGIC EVENTS IN SPORTS

On March 22, 1989, Clint Malarchuck, the goalie for the Buffalo Sabres, was struck in the neck by the skate of opponent Steve Tuttle, slicing his jugular vein. He lost an estimated 1.5 L of blood before athletic trainer Jim Pizzutelli was able to apply pressure to the wound and stop the bleeding. He required 300 sutures and was back to playing in 10 days.

On February 10, 2008, Richard Zednik of the Florida Panthers was playing against the Buffalo Sabres when his teammate Olli Jokinen collided with Saber player Clarke MacArther. During the collision, Zednik's carotid artery was severed by Jokinen's skate. Zednik lost an estimated 2 L of blood. The team's athletic trainer, Dave Zenobi, applied pressure to stop the bleeding until they arrived at DeRay Medical Center.

disease may not be able to adapt to this reduction-relative anemia and myocardial infarction may result. A myocardial infarction causes cardiogenic shock, further decreasing the circulating blood volume and exacerbating the shock state. The patient now suffers from hypovolemic shock and cardiogenic shock. Treatment for these may include volume replacement via fluids, blood, or blood products, and a combination of alpha- and beta-adrenergic agents.

Distributive Shock

Distributive shock is a broad category of shock in which blood or its components will be unevenly distributed throughout the vasculature, resulting in poor perfusion to tissues and vital organs. Consider sepsis, which causes dilation and increased permeability of the capillary beds, allowing plasma to leak into the intracellular spaces. The result is edema, decreased systemic vascular resistance, inability of oxygen to cross the cellular membranes, and, eventually, cellular death. The cell walls of Gram-negative bacteria, such as *Escherichia coli*, *Klebsiella*, and *Proteus*, contain lipopolysaccharide that causes additional physiological complications. Release of lipopolysaccharide into the circulation on bacterial cell death causes damage to the pulmonary capillaries, resulting in disseminated intravascular coagulation. This compounds the effects of decreased perfusion and increases the risk of mortality.

Neurogenic shock is similar to anaphylactic shock, as both are the result of severe vasodilation but the mechanisms are very different. Neurogenic shock is caused by an insult to the descending sympathetic tracts of the spinal cord above the sixth thoracic vertebrae. This disruption of sympathetic tone allows the parasympathetic tone to dominate. Generalized vasodilation and shock immediately result. The effect may be temporary, if caused by a hematoma or contusion, but it may be extensive in the event of spinal cord disruption.

Cardiogenic Shock

Cardiogenic shock results from decreased cardiac output. Some causes include cardiac dysrhythmias, myocardial infarction, ruptured heart valves, and cardiac contusion. Cardiac dysrhythmias disrupt the well-choreographed action of the cardiac cycle. They can decrease the preload to the ventricles (as in atrial fibrillation), result in inability of the ventricle to adequately fill (as in supraventricular tachycardia), or decrease minute volume due to bradycardia from lower heart block. Myocardial infarctions are blockages of the major coronary arteries by plaque or thromboses, causing ischemia or death to the affected myocardium. The

Table 8-2. Signs and Symptoms of Shock		
Sign	Compensated Shock	Uncompensated Shock
Heart rate	Mildly increased	Markedly increased
Skin	Normal to cool	Cool, pale, clammy
Mental status	Normal	Dizzy, syncope, unconscious
Respirations	Normal	Tachypnea
Blood pressure	Normal	Decreased

extent of the damage, and thus severity of shock, depends on the size of the affected area and the specific myocardial tissue involved. For example, occlusions of the right heart are generally less devastating than those involving the left heart. The left anterior descending artery supplies the left ventricle and septum and, if occluded, is called the *widow-maker* because it often results in sudden cardiac death.

Obstructive Shock

Although sometimes classified as cardiogenic shock due to location, obstructive shock is differentiated by the physical obstruction of the heart or great vessels. Similar to cardiogenic shock, obstructive shock results in reduced cardiac output—not from a cardiac dysfunction, but rather from a direct restriction of blood flow.

One example of an obstructive event leading to shock is cardiac tamponade. This occurs when fluid—often blood—collects within the pericardial sac, thereby compressing the heart. As the tamponade accumulates and cardiac output decreases, the pulse pressure narrows and shock ensues. Another example is pulmonary embolism, which is the result of a thrombus or air bubble that lodges in the pulmonary vasculature. This prevents gas exchange in the lung tissue distal to this blockage. The degree of shock is directly proportional to the size of the vessel that is blocked. Another example is a tension pneumothorax. Similar to cardiac tamponade, a tension pneumothorax occurs when air is trapped in the pleural space. The affected lung is compressed as the volume of air increases. This decreases the number of alveoli for gas exchange. When the amount of unoxygenated blood being shunted to the left heart reaches a critical level, hypoxia develops. In addition, the unilateral increased intrathoracic pressure displaces the mediastinum, kinks the aortic arch, and severely decreases the cardiac output.

Signs and Symptoms of Shock

Rapid assessment and intervention are the keys to successful resuscitation of an individual in shock. Recognition of early signs and symptoms can help the athletic trainer intervene early and avoid the rapid escalation of the cascading events leading to decompensation and death. These early signals are not always obvious, and identifying them is more of an art than a science.

As the patient transitions from normal hemodynamic perfusion to hemodynamic instability due to shock, he or she will, at least briefly, compensate for the shock. For example, if an athlete loses fluid due to dehydration, the body will initially compensate for mild fluid loss by increasing the heart rate, vasoconstriction, and cardiac contractility. These measures can compensate temporarily and arrest the progression of shock if the underlying condition is corrected. Therefore, if rehydration is started and fluid is replaced, progress to shock is halted. However, if, the underlying condition is not corrected or is allowed to worsen, the body's compensatory mechanisms become overwhelmed and shock ensues.

Hypovolemic shock is the most common type of shock encountered by the athletic trainer. Signs and symptoms of compensated hypovolemic shock are dry mucous membranes, thirst, decreased urination, concentrated urine, and mild tachycardia. Blood pressure is ultimately maintained. As shock progresses and compensatory mechanisms are unable to cope with the fluid deficit, signs and symptoms become associated with hypoperfusion syndrome. The body defenses shunt fluid away from the periphery to preserve the brain, heart, and kidneys. Thus, signs and symptoms of uncompensated shock include pale, clammy skin; weak, thready pulse; tachycardia; lightheadedness; syncope; and hypotension. When these developments occur, the vital organs begin to suffer from lack of perfusion. If corrective action is not taken, the risk of permanent injury to these organs increases (Table 8-2).

Sepsis

When the body is invaded by microorganisms, it responds in a predictable manner. This response involves attacking the microbes by increasing production of and dispatching leukocytes (white blood cells) to the infected areas. Leukocytes engulf and immobilize organisms, clearing them from the body. Some microorganisms and parasites have developed their own defenses, by which they use the leukocytes as hosts or transport vessels, thus evading the leukocyte system of defense.

TABLE 8-3. MRSA SURVIVABILITY

SURFACE	LIFESPAN
Dust	7 months
Mop head	8 weeks
Cotton towel	9 weeks
Blanket	6 months

The body also battles invading organisms through isolation. Walls of fluid and immune cells surround the invaders locally, thus preventing widespread and overwhelming infection. This walling-off isolation forms septic cysts. Although the organisms are still alive, they are contained locally and are unable to cause whole-body effects. For example, with boils or abscesses, the body walls off or encapsulates the infection in an effort to prevent its dissemination.

Common symptoms of infections, which may vary by causative agent, include fever, chills, inflammation, and leukocytosis. As the body's defenses become overwhelmed, hypotension, lethargy, and septic shock may develop. If extrinsic intervention is not employed, the shock state worsens, and severe illness or death results. Rapid diagnosis; treatment with effective antibiotics or antiviral agents, intravenous fluids, and vasopressors; and systemic support may be needed until infectious organisms are eradicated.

Although these microbes can also be fungi, yeasts, or parasites, they are most frequently bacterial or viral. They can be acquired from sources that include contact with surfaces such as floors, mats, and equipment; water from saunas and whirlpools; other individuals, such as skin contact or bodily secretions; or with insect vectors, such as mosquitos or ticks. Resulting infections can be as simple as upper respiratory and skin infections or as serious as blood and bone infections.

Management of infection in the athletic training environment can be cumbersome. Most sports involve contact with some or all of these modes of transmission. Infectious disease outbreaks are becoming more frequent. In a study done by Collins and O'Connell, 57% of the reported infectious disease outbreaks in Ireland were at the high school and collegiate level.[1]

Staphylococcus Aureus

Species of *Staphylococcus* are some of the most resilient, non–spore-forming bacteria. *Staphylococcus aureus* are commonly found in the nasal openings or nares of 30% to 40% of the population. When living on our bodies, these organisms are relatively harmless. However, they are opportunistic and can cause infection via a disruption of the integrity of the skin. These skin disruptions (eg,

scratches, abrasions, lacerations, and hair follicles) provide a portal of entry through the otherwise impenetrable layers of our skin. When entrenched, *S. aureus* can cause localized infection by forming subcutaneous, deep tissue, or bone abscesses. With an impressive array of virulence factors, it can invade the underlying muscle, tendons, ligaments, and bone and even destroy tissue or bone. Other routes of infection of *S. aureus* are inhalation, resulting in pneumonia, and blood stream infection, which can result in generalized or overwhelming sepsis.

S. aureus is transmitted by direct contact with other individuals or by contact with surfaces that have been colonized. *S. aureus* can survive from a few days to 7 months, especially on nonporous surfaces.[2] The duration of survival on surfaces depends on factors that include temperature and humidity[3] (Table 8-3).

Methicillin-Resistant Staphylococcus Aureus

S. aureus was first isolated in the 1880s. Decades of overuse and misuse of the antibiotic penicillin has allowed antibiotic resistances to emerge in *S. aureus*. Methicillin, a different type of antibiotic, was developed to combat penicillin-resistant strains. In the 1940s and 1950s, *S. aureus* strains also developed resistance to methicillin and the entire group of beta-lactam antibiotics.[4] Resistant infections were first observed in athletes in the 1960s, but it was not until 1993 that the first outbreak involving 6 high school wrestlers was documented. Initially, methicillin-resistant *S. aureus* (MRSA) was seen almost exclusively in people who had contact with the health care system—hence the term *healthcare–acquired MRSA*. Since then, it unfortunately has become more prevalent and is also recognized as community-acquired MRSA.

Most MRSA sports outbreaks have been associated with contact sports such as rugby, soccer, wrestling, volleyball, and, especially, football. MRSA is now commonly found to be in the nares of many healthy people, but it does not cause infection unless it finds an opportunity. MRSA can also live on environmental surfaces for long periods of time[5] (Table 8-3). Waninger et al[6] found that MRSA embedded in artificial turf can likely live indefinitely if provided with nutrients such as mucin, which is found in nasal secretions and saliva.

MRSA presents with painful, erythemic lesions that are often associated with fever, chills, and fatigue, and almost all antibiotics are ineffective at eliminating these bacteria. Small infections can often be treated with warm compresses and antibiotics. However, these infections progress rapidly and frequently require incision and drainage, with or without the addition of antimicrobial agents such as clindamycin, doxycycline, or trimethoprim-sulfamethoxazole. It is important to note antibiotic side effects. For example, doxycycline can predispose individuals to first-degree sunburn; therefore, it should be used cautiously in athletes involved in outdoor sports.

Tetanus

Tetanus is a rare but very serious infection, with a 20% mortality rate. It is a non communicable bacterial infection caused by the microorganism *Clostridium tetani*. Spores of these bacteria are most prevalent in soil and dust and can be acquired when infected dirt or dust enters an opening in the skin, such as from a puncture wound (eg, stepping on a nail or piece of glass). When embedded in an oxygen-depleted environment, *C. tetani* spores become active cells again, rapidly reproducing and excreting neurotoxins. These neurotoxins cause a bone-breaking contraction of muscles, and the spasms are indicative of tetanus. The classic muscle spasms of the jaw led to the disease becoming commonly known as *lockjaw*.

Tetanus is easily preventable by vaccination with DTaP, a vaccine for diphtheria, tetanus, and pertussis, or whooping cough. It contains inactivated toxins, called *toxoids*, to mount immunity to diphtheria and tetanus toxins by the body, and it contains an acellular component of the bacterium that causes pertussis, also stimulating immunity. However this immunity does not last a lifetime, and boosters are required to maintain immunity. The Centers for Disease Control and Prevention immunization schedule for children and adolescents aged 18 years and younger in the United States recommends DTaP at 2, 4, 6, and 15 months, followed by periodic boosters every 10 years to maintain protection against these 3 diseases.

The Centers for Disease Control and Prevention estimates that only 84.6% of infants aged 19 to 35 months in the United States have received the recommended 4 doses of DTaP/TDaP immunizations.[7] This means that more than 15% of children may be susceptible to tetanus neurotoxins. Therefore, it is important for athletic trainers to be diligent with wound cleansing and follow-up recommendations for all athletes who have sustained open wounds, but especially those who have not had their childhood immunizations.

Fungal Infections

Other less-concerning infections include localized fungal infections such as athlete's foot (tinea pedis), ringworm (tinea corporis), and jock itch (tinea cruris). These are easily spread from athlete to athlete due to the warm, moist environment of gyms and locker rooms. In addition, these fungi, termed *dermatophytes*, can be harbored on and acquired from mats, floors, shared towels, and pools. In 2005, according to the National Collegiate Athletic Association, fungal infections accounted for 22% of all dermatologic infections among college wrestlers.[8]

Herpes Simplex Virus Type 1

Herpes simplex virus 1 is commonly spread through direct skin-to-skin contact. Primary lesions initially present as fluid-filled vesicles that develop into ulcerations upon bursting. They are most commonly seen on or around the lips, oral cavity or buccal membranes, and the tongue, as the virus travels up and down the facial nerves. The lesions are often preceded by local pain and fever, followed by pain and swelling of the submandibular and cervical lymph nodes in the jaw and neck. Recurrent infections more frequently present as clusters of lesions rather than singular lesions. Although recurrent infections are frequently found in and around the oral cavity, they can erupt anywhere, including the head, hands, toes, and fingers.

Because herpes simplex virus 1 is a lifelong condition, the virus is never eradicated but is merely suppressed for periods of time by the immune system. Therefore, when to return to active sports is always a concern after an outbreak (Table 8-4).

Anaphylaxis

When the body is initially exposed to an allergy-inducing compound, the immune system develops antibodies to combat these specific allergens during future exposures. Mild allergic reactions can cause local irritation, rash, sinus congestion, watery eyes, and pruritis. These responses are generally self-limiting and can be managed with antihistamines and other topical medications. More severe immune reactions can cause bronchoconstriction, vasodilation, increased capillary permeability, and tachycardia. These reactions may be managed with antihistamines, systemic steroids, intravenous fluids, and supportive care.

Anaphylactic shock is dangerous and is caused by the body's exaggerated immune response to an allergen. When an allergen to which an individual has hypersensitivity enters the body and bloodstream, the body reacts by producing histamines, kinins, and prostaglandins. Vasodilation and increased capillary permeability occur, similar to other types of shock, but the constriction of extravascular smooth muscle causes severe bronchoconstriction. This results in the hallmark wheezing and air hunger associated with anaphylaxis, and bronchoconstriction exacerbates the already-decreased oxygen delivery to the cells. Vasodilation leads to edema and hypovolemia-like symptoms. Left uncorrected, hypoxia and hypotension worsen until cellular anoxia leads to cell death and damage or death of vital organs. This condition is life-threatening and can occur rapidly in some cases.

Initial management includes supplemental oxygen, oral or intravenous fluids, antihistamines, steroids, and intramuscular injection of epinephrine. Epinephrine, a hormone and a neurotransmitter, can be given as a 1-mg injection or delivered as a prefilled EpiPen (Mylan Specialty LP). Epinephrine acts as both a bronchodilator and vasoconstrictor, thus increasing respirations as well as correcting hypotension. The effects of the injection last about 15 minutes, after which symptoms may return. Therefore, supportive care and rapid transport to a medical facility are essential for the best outcome.

TABLE 8-4. HERPES SIMPLEX VIRUS-1 RETURN TO ACTIVE-SPORTS CRITERIA

TYPE OF INFECTION	NATIONAL COLLEGIATE ATHLETIC ASSOCIATION*[9]	NATIONAL FEDERATION OF STATE HIGH SCHOOL ASSOCIATIONS[10]
Primary	1. Free of systemic symptoms of viral infection 2. No new blisters for 72 hours 3. No moist lesions; lesions must be dry and surmounted by a firm, adherent crust 4. Antivirals for 120 hours 5. Not be covered to participate	The infected individual must be immediately removed from contact and seek appropriate care and treatment. Return to contact is permissible only after all lesions are healed with well-adherent scabs, no new vesicles have formed, and no swollen lymph nodes remain in the affected area.
Recurrent	1. No moist lesions; lesions must be dry and surmounted by a firm, adherent crust 2. Antivirals for 120 hours 3. Not be covered to participate	If antivirals, no contact for 5 days
* Wrestling regulations		

Exercise-Induced Anaphylaxis

Exercise-induced anaphylaxis (EIA), first described in 1979,[11] is a clinical condition that happens when anaphylaxis occurs in combination with physical activity. Initially, it was thought to be related to ingestion of food allergens, specifically shellfish, prior to exercise. Du Toit[12] estimated that 5% to 15% of anaphylactic reactions are associated with exercise—independent of prior food intake—and this view is now widely accepted. EIA occurs in all ages and is most common in those whose exercise is suboptimal. It occurs in professional athletes as well as beginners. Activities such as jogging, running, cycling, basketball, soccer, and swimming are among the sports most prominently associated with EIA.[13]

EIA seems to be triggered by mast cell production during exercise. Mast cells are a normal component of our immune systems and release histamines and other allergy-triggering molecules. This cascade of events results in classic symptoms of anaphylaxis such as flushing of the skin, urticaria (hives), angioedema, wheezing, bronchospasms, and laryngeal edema.

Acute management of EIA, like acute management of anaphylaxis of other causes, is critical and follows the same treatments. Epinephrine injection via either weight-based administration or prefilled autoinjector is the most rapid and effective treatment. Notably, epinephrine has a half-life of 2 to 4 minutes, meaning that only half of the administered dose is functioning at 2 to 4 minutes post-injection. Immediate transport to a medical facility is essential for longer term management because the patient may relapse with symptoms as the drug is metabolized. Other tools for preventative management include histamine blockers such as diphenhydramine and famotidine.

The primary obligation of the athletic trainer is treating and preventing musculoskeletal injuries; however, other emergencies and other factors can affect the athlete's health and performance. Shock can occur for a variety of reasons, and the athletic trainer is the on-scene person who can make the difference between a manageable emergency and a catastrophic event. Anaphylaxis too can be managed if identified early and managed appropriately. In addition to on-field situations, disease prevention and treatment can ensure that athletes are healthy, their exposure to disease is minimized, and their availability to participate is maximized. The old adage, "An ounce of prevention is worth a pound of cure," is true for athletic injuries and illnesses. But, when prevention is not enough, preparing for the multitude of potential events can make all the difference in the world.

CHAPTER SUMMARY

Orthopedic and musculoskeletal injuries have traditionally been the major emphasis of athletic trainers and other members of the sports medicine community. However, this paradigm has changed. The athletic trainer now is part of the health care community and plays a more comprehensive role in the athlete's overall wellness. Athletic trainers must be versed in immunizations, communicable diseases and disease prevention, infection control and management, and recognition and management of other serious or life-threatening situations such as shock, asthma, and anaphylaxis. Their role has become more complex and demanding and will, undoubtedly, continue to evolve and expand. The knowledge base of the athletic trainer must evolve and expand as well.

CHAPTER REVIEW QUESTIONS

1. What is the common result of all types of shock?
2. How does anaphylaxis differ from a simple allergic reaction?
3. True or false: MRSA can survive only on living tissue.
4. True or false: Tetanus can be passed from person to person through sweat or saliva.
5. What is the difference between compensated and uncompensated shock?

ANSWERS

1. Inadequate perfusion of vital organs.
2. Anaphylactic shock is an exaggerated response to an allergen.
3. False. MRSA can survive on inanimate surfaces for an extended period of time.
4. False. Tetanus is not a communicable disease.
5. Patients with uncompensated shock can no longer maintain viable vital signs and have a weak pulse and hypotension.

REFERENCES

1. Collins C, O'Connell B. Infectious disease outbreaks in competitive sports, 2005-2010. *J Athl Train*. 2012;47(5):516-18.
2. Kramer A, Schwebke I, Kampf G. How long do nosocomial pathogens last on inanimate surfaces? A systematic review. *BMC Infectious Disease*. 2006;6:130.
3. Neely A, Maley M. Survival of enterococci and staphylococci on hospital fabrics and plastics. *J Clin Microbiol*. 2000; 38(2):724-26.
4. National Institute of Allergy and Infectious Diseases, National Institutes of Health, United States. *History, methicillin-resistant Staphylococcus aureus, Antimicrobial Resistance*. 2016. https://www.niaid.nih.gov/research/mrsa-antimicrobial-resistance-history. Accessed May 14, 2018.
5. Millersville University. Questions About MRSA. http://www.millersville.edu/athletictraining/mrsa/faq.php. Accessed May 14, 2018.
6. Waninger KN, Rooney TP, Miller JE, Berberian J, Fujimoto A, Buttaro BA. Community-associated methicillin-resistant *Staphylococcus aureus* survival on artificial turf substrates. *Med Sci Sports Exerc*. 2011;43(5):779-84.
7. Centers for Disease Control and Prevention. FastStats - Immunization. https://www.cdc.gov/nchs/fastats/immunize.htm. Accessed May 18, 2018.
8. Shah N, Cain G, Naji O, Goff J. Skin infections in athletes: treating the patient, protecting the team. *J Fam Pract*. 2013;(26)284-91.
9. Zinder S, Basler R, et al *National Athletic Trainers' Association Position Statement: Skin Diseases*. https://www.ncbi.nlm.nih.gov/pmc/articles/PMC2902037/ Accessed August 5, 2018.
10. The National Federation of State High School Associations. Sports-related skin infections position statement and guidelines. https://www.nfhs.org/media/1014740/sports_related_skin_infections_position_statement_and_guidelines_-final-april-2018.pdf. Accessed August 5, 2018.
11. Maulitz RM, Pratt DA, Schocket AL. Exercise-induced anaphylactic reaction to shellfish. *J Allergy Clin Immunol*. 1979;63:433-434.
12. Du Toit G. Food-dependent exercise-induced anaphylaxis in childhood. *Pediatr Child Immunol*. 2007;18:455-463.
13. Castells MC, Horan RF, Sheffer AL. Exercise-induced anaphylaxis. *Curr Allergy Asthma Rep*. 2003;(3)15-21.

9

Wound Management and Bleeding Control

Alan Shapiro, DO

CHAPTER KEY WORDS

- Bleeding
- Skin
- Trauma

CHAPTER SCENARIO

An 18-year-old male high school soccer player collides with another player while going for the ball. The other player's spike strikes the first player's anterior medial tibia region. He sustains obvious bruising and a laceration. The player asks the athletic trainer to butterfly it closed so he can continue to play the game.

SCENARIO RESOLUTION

The athletic trainer determines that due to the depth and appearance of the wound, it would not be amenable to a butterfly bandage. It has deep portions and needs appropriate wound care that cannot be provided on site. The athletic trainer appropriately applies a dry dressing and refers the patient to the local emergency department for definitive care. In the emergency department the patient has the wound cleansed with Hibiclens (chlorhexidine gluconate) solution. The wound bed is then anesthetized with lidocaine with epinephrine. The dermal avulsion is pulled back, and the wound is copiously irrigated. There is no evidence of tendon or ligament injury or exposed bone. The avulsed tissue is approximated as best as possible. The deep layers are approximated with absorbable suture, then the superficial layers are closed using a running nylon suture. The wound is dressed with antibiotic ointment, a nonadherent dressing, gauze, and kling. Daily dressing changes are performed. On day 10, the sutures are removed without complication.

INTRODUCTION

Patients can sustain injuries to their skin and underlying structures from direct and/or indirect injury, as well as blunt and/or penetrating trauma. This chapter will focus on basic anatomy of the integumentary system and its underlying components, common injuries, and life-threatening injuries. The basic principles of wound care will be discussed, and control of hemorrhage will be explained.

Skin

The skin is the largest organ of the human body and comprises the integumentary system, which protects the underlying muscles, bones, ligaments, and internal organs. The skin is composed of 3 layers: the epidermis, dermis, and hypodermis (Figure 9-1).

Feld F., Gorse KM, Blanc RO
Non–Orthopedic Emergency Care in Athletics (pp 65-73).
© 2020 Taylor & Francis Group.

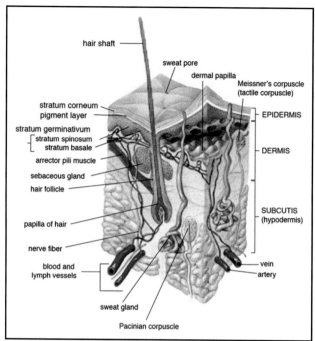

Figure 9-1. Anatomy of the skin.

Epidermis

The epidermis is the outermost layer, which forms a protective barrier over the body surface. The epidermis helps regulate body temperature and contains no blood vessels.

Dermis

The dermis is the layer underneath the epidermis and consists of connective tissue that cushions the body from stress and strain. The dermis is tightly connected to the epidermis and contains nerve endings, blood vessels, lymphatic vessels, hair follicles, and exocrine glands. The dermis is divided into 2 regions. The papillary region comprises areolar connective tissue. The papillae extend toward the epidermis and provide the dermis with a rough surface that integrates with the epidermis, which strengthens the connections between the two layers of skin. The reticular region lies deep in the papillary region and contains dense irregular connective tissue that contains collagen, elastin, and reticular fibers.

Hypodermis

The hypodermis is the subcutaneous tissue that lies below the dermis and consists of adipose tissue and elastin. The hypodermis attaches the dermis to the underlying muscle and bone and contains nerves and blood vessels.

Trauma to the Skin

Skin injuries can be sustained through direct or indirect contact and can be caused by both penetrating and non-penetrating sources. Common traumatic injuries include contusions, abrasions, penetrating injuries, burns, and lacerations.[1]

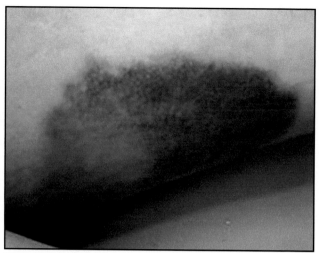

Figure 9-2. Contusion.

Contusions

Contusions are regions of skin in which the capillaries have been ruptured. Contusions will go through evolutionary stages until they resolve. They can be painful, and, depending on the nature of the injury, there could be concern for underlying trauma. Treatment for isolated contusions includes rest, ice, and elevation of the extremity. They can take days to weeks to resolve. Contusions should be monitored to ensure they are resolving and that a hematoma is not expanding under the skin (Figure 9-2).

Abrasions

Abrasions are wounds caused by superficial damage to the epidermis. Abrasions involve contact with an object or surface and can be superficial or deep. Superficial abrasions heal without scarring, whereas deep abrasions can form scar tissue. Abrasions usually bleed at the time of injury and can be painful. Treatment for abrasions includes washing the affected area with soap and water and removing any debris from the wound bed. They should be covered with antibiotic ointment and a nonadherent dressing and then wrapped with gauze and Curlex (American Excelsior Company). This should be done at least once or twice per day, and the area should be monitored for signs of infection (Figure 9-3).

Burns

Burns are common household and industrial injuries. They can be caused by liquids, chemicals, fire, electricity, inhalation, and ultraviolet radiation. Burns are characterized based on severity of damage to the skin and on depth. The current classification system references superficial (first-degree), partial-thickness (second-degree), and full-thickness (third-degree) burns. Burns to the face, hands,

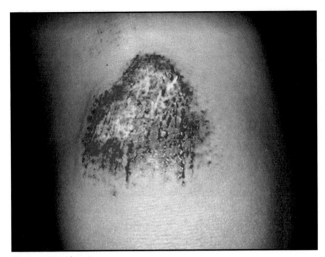

Figure 9-3. Abrasion.

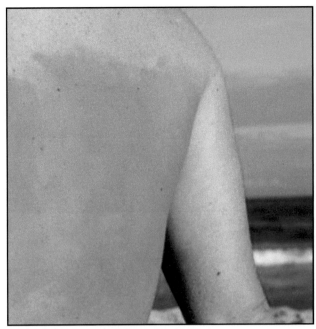

Figure 9-4. Superficial burn.

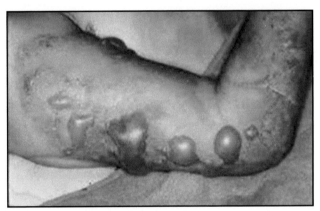

Figure 9-5. Superficial partial-thickness burn.

and genitals are considered critical burns. Any partial- or full-thickness burn in a child with greater than 10% body surface area affected or an adult with greater than 15% to 20% of the body's body surface area affected is considered significant and should be evaluated at a burn/trauma center.

Sunburn

Sunburn is an inflammatory response that causes damage to DNA in the skin cells as a result of overexposure to ultraviolet radiation. Typically, the skin becomes reddened, hot, with or without mild swelling, and can be associated with pain and fatigue. Certain populations, including children and the elderly, can be especially susceptible, and preventative measures, such as using sunscreen, are helpful. Sunburn is a superficial burn that can be treated with moisturizing cream.

Superficial (First-Degree) Burns

Superficial burns usually affect the epidermis. The site of injury appears red, painful, and dry, without blister formation. Superficial burns usually resolve with conservative treatment, and long-term tissue damage is rare (Figure 9-4).

Partial-Thickness (Second-Degree) Burns

Partial-thickness burns involve the epidermis and part of the dermis. The site of injury appears red, swollen, and painful, with blister formation. Partial-thickness burns can be further classified into superficial and deep partial-thickness burns, depending on the degree of the dermis involved. Fluid will build up under the skin and separate the epidermis from the dermis. When the blister ruptures, it will expose the dermis, and, depending on the total body surface area involved, significant water loss and loss of thermoregulation can occur. Caution must be taken when managing partial-thickness burns, as they can evolve into full-thickness burns despite treatment. Partial-thickness burns require treatment by a certified burn/trauma physician and, depending on the percent body surface area and

depth, may require skin grafting. Smaller partial-thickness burns will heal by contracting scarring. These burns, if untreated, can lead to hypothermia, infection, sepsis, and death (Figure 9-5).

Full-Thickness (Third-Degree) Burns

Full thickness burns involve the epidermis and the dermis. They can also involve the underlying muscle, tendon, and bone. The site of injury is white and leathery or can appear charred. These burns are insensate, as the nerve endings are damaged. Full-thickness burns require treatment by a certified burn/trauma physician and, depending on the percent body surface area, will require skin grafting. Smaller full-thickness burns will heal by contracting scarring. These burns, if untreated, can lead to hypothermia, infection, sepsis, and death (Figure 9-6).

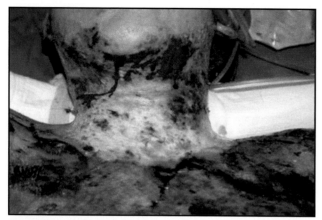

Figure 9-6. Full-thickness burn.

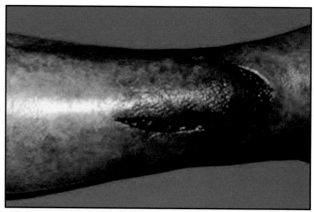

Figure 9-7. Avulsion laceration.

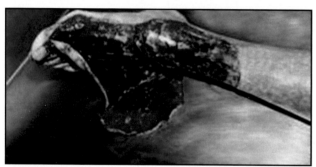

Figure 9-8. Extensive laceration and degloving injury of a patient's foot and ankle.

Treatment of Burns

Treatment of burns involves stopping the burning process, which can be accomplished by removing the patient from the environment or the process from the patient. However, ensure your safety first. All partial- and full-thickness burns should be covered with a dry dressing, and the patient should be transported to a facility capable of handling burn patients. Prior to handling the burn injuries, the patient should be assessed for any other threats to life.

Lacerations

Lacerations are common injuries that involve contact with an object or surface that causes damage through the epidermis and dermis, with a superficial or deep break in the skin. Lacerations can involve the fatty tissue below the hypodermis, tendons, ligaments, and muscle and can expose bone. Lacerations are classified based on location, length, and depth. Lacerations involving the fingers, toes, and joints must be evaluated for tendon and nerve injury distal to the site and may require subspecialist consultation to evaluate and repair the underlying damage. Lacerations over major blood vessels and arteries should be evaluated for vascular injury, and, if one is found, consultation with the appropriate subspecialist may be necessary. Lacerations can occur over fractures, and fractures can also injure the

tissues and protrude through the skin. Lacerations may cause pain and discomfort as well (Figures 9-7 and 9-8).[2]

Treatment of Lacerations

Treatment of lacerations involves controlling any active bleeding site. When the bleeding is controlled, the wound should be dressed with a dry, sterile dressing. The wound will need to be evaluated for depth, foreign debris, irrigation or wash out, and closure.

Prior to wound closure, the wound should be cleansed with an antimicrobial skin cleanser. Chlorhexidine is a broad-spectrum antimicrobial skin cleanser and antiseptic. It provides long-lasting antimicrobial activity. Then, after cleaning, the affected area can be anesthetized, using a local anesthetic such as Xylocaine (lidocaine), with or without epinephrine. Epinephrine should be avoided in the distal extremities and in any tissue where there is poor vascular supply. Betadine (povidone-iodine), hydrogen peroxide, and alcohol will kill bacteria, but they can also cause irritation to healthy tissue and the wound bed; thus, these agents should be avoided in open wounds.

There are several methods of closing a wound. Location, depth, risk of underlying injury, and infection are all of concern and may contribute to how the wound is closed. Any wound in which there is debris must be copiously irrigated and washed out prior to closure. All lacerations should be closed within 8 hours of injury, as the further treatment is delayed, the more opportunity infection has to occur. However, this needs to be evaluated on a case-by-case basis, depending on the mechanism of injury, site of injury, and degree of tissue damage. Delayed closure is an option; however, it should be reserved for the wounds that are most likely to become infected.

Closure options include dermal adhesives, Steri-Strip (Nexcare) wound closures, stitches, and staples. Dermal adhesives are an excellent choice for a clean, nonbleeding, superficial, small wound. Steri-Strip closures are an alternative to dermal adhesives, but are not a substitute for stitches and staples, which should be used for deeper and longer wounds, or wounds where there is a greater chance of dehiscence or injury. Deep wounds may require multiple-layer closure, in which the deep sutures should be absorbable. Nonabsorbable sutures and staples will need to be removed after a period of time, depending on the location and degree of injury.

For cosmetic purposes, stitches will offer the best wound-edge approximation, closure, and minimized scarring. Staples are an excellent choice for scalp wounds and some post-surgical wounds, as they are made of titanium or stainless steel, which lessens the reaction with the immune system. All wounds, regardless of the method of closure, will heal with a scar. Scars can be revised should they not be to the patient's liking or form a keloid, which is an overgrowth of scar tissue.

When a wound is closed, it should be washed with soap and water at least once daily, and then either an antibiotic ointment or non-petroleum based, non-scented, non-alcohol–containing moisturizing cream should be applied. The wound should be inspected daily for signs of infection, including redness, purulence, swelling, and pain. If the wound is over a joint, it may require short-term immobilization to prevent damage to the wound bed while it heals. Splinting should be used with caution to prevent joint stiffening, muscle atrophy, and loss of function. If underlying tendon, ligament, or muscle is involved, the patient should be splinted in a position of function, with appropriate referral to a specialist for definitive care. If there is an obvious fracture exposed through a wound, a dry dressing and splint should be applied, and the patient should be transported to a facility capable of handling open fractures.

Penetrating Injuries

Penetrating trauma can occur as a result of any object puncturing the skin and entering a body, creating an open wound. The most common penetrating injuries are lacerations; others include stab wounds, gunshot wounds, and impalements. Any penetrating injury needs to be assessed based on location, mechanism of injury, and the potential vascular structures and organs underlying the site of injury. If the penetrating object is impaled in the patient, it should not be removed until potential underlying injury has been ruled out. The only caveat would be in a patient who could not be moved or transported safety due to the object. If the trauma is a stab wound or gunshot, focus should be aimed at hemorrhage control and getting the patient to definitive care.[3,4]

All patients, regardless of the site of injury or mechanism of injury, should initially be evaluated using the ABCDE method: Airway, Breathing, Circulation, Disability, and Exposure.

- **Airway**: Does the patient have an airway? If not, and there is no suspected cervical spine injury, open the airway using a head tilt, chin lift. If there is suspected cervical spine injury, a jaw thrust or tongue jaw lift should be used.

- **Breathing**: Is the patient breathing? If the patient is breathing, is the breathing effective and adequate? If the breathing is inadequate, the patient may require supplemental oxygen, rescue breathing, or ventilation with a bag-valve mask.
- **Circulation**: Does the patient have a pulse? If not, cardiopulmonary resuscitation should be initiated. If the patient has a pulse, assess whether it is strong or weak and regular or irregular. A weak, fast pulse can be an ominous sign of shock, whereas a strong pulse can indicate adequate blood pressure and tissue perfusion.
- **Disability**: When vital function has been assessed, locate the site or sites of disability or injury.
- **Exposure**: Expose the site of disability or injury. This will allow you to adequately assess the site and institute the appropriate care.

For penetrating injuries to the head, neck, chest, abdomen, and pelvis in which there is internal bleeding, this cannot be controlled outside the hospital. The emergency management services system should be activated, and the patient should be transported to the closest appropriate facility. Care must also be taken when evaluating the neck and chest for penetrating trauma.

Head

The head contains the brain, eyes, upper airways, and facial structures. Blunt or penetrating injury can be life-threatening, especially in the case of intracranial bleeding. Any patient with a blunt or penetrating head injury—with or without mental status change, site threatening injury, or airway compromise—should be promptly transported to the closest appropriate facility.

Neck

The neck contains the external and internal jugular veins as well as external and internal carotid arteries. Direct pressure is best to control bleeding from these vessels; however, an exsanguinating hemorrhage can occur quickly if not identified and treated promptly. The trachea, if lacerated, can cause respiratory distress, failure, and subcutaneous emphysema. This represents an airway and surgical emergency (Figure 9-9).

Chest

The chest contains the heart, aorta, vena cava, lungs, trachea, esophagus, and other great vessels. If not identified and treated quickly, internal injury to any of these organs and vessels can be significant. Any injury to the heart, aorta, other great vessels, or vena cava can lead to exsanguination in the chest cavity. Penetrating or blunt injury to the chest can cause a pneumothorax, hemothorax, or hemopneumothorax.

Pneumothorax (Figure 9-10) is when air leaks into the pleural cavity and causes the lung to collapse. Tension pneumothorax is when the trachea deviates to the side

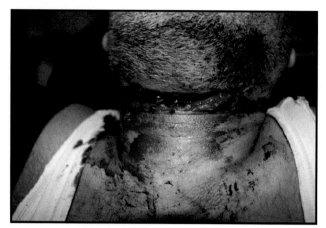

Figure 9-9. Penetrating neck injury.

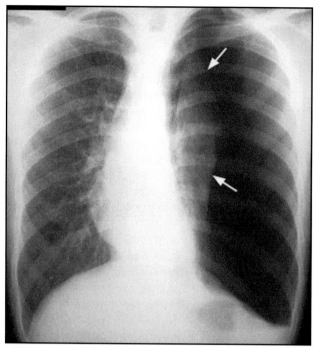

Figure 9-10. Left-sided pneumothorax.

opposite the pneumothorax. A hemothorax is when blood is in the pleural cavity. A hemopneumothorax is when air and blood are in the pleural space. A patient who has a suspected pneumothorax or tension pneumothorax should have a trained provider perform a needle decompression at either the second intercostal space at the mid-clavicular line or fourth intercostal space mid-axillary line. Definitive care includes a thoracostomy tube to allow for lung reexpansion and/or drainage of the hemothorax. If the hemothorax is significant or the bleeding persists, the patient may require an operative intervention to control the hemorrhage and repair any underlying damaged vessels and/or organs.

Abdomen and Pelvis

The abdomen and pelvis contain the liver, spleen, kidneys, stomach, small bowel, colon, pancreas, gall bladder, appendix, aorta, inferior vena cava, iliac vessels, ureters, and bladder. In women, the pelvis also contains the uterus, ovaries, and fallopian tubes. All of these can be injured by blunt or penetrating trauma. Internal injury to the vasculature, liver, kidneys, and spleen can lead to life-threatening hemorrhage. Injury to the other organs can lead to complications if not treated promptly. In the event of an evisceration, in which the contents of the abdomen are outside of the abdominal cavity, they should be covered with a dry sterile dressing that is moistened with sterile water or saline.

Extremities

Injuries to the extremities can range from minor to severe. Bleeding can be minor or life-threatening. After airway, breathing, and circulation have been assessed and managed, and the disability has been exposed and identified, hemorrhage control is of paramount importance. Part of controlling hemorrhage might involve applying a splint to stabilize the extremity injury, applying a tourniquet, or packing the wound.

Hemorrhage Control/Stop the Bleed

Stop the Bleed is a national awareness campaign and call to action. The program is intended to encourage bystanders to become trained, equipped, and empowered to help in an emergency prior to the arrival of professional help. This program has applicability to both the lay rescuer and the professional rescuer or health care professional.[5-11]

Any victim of trauma, whether blunt or penetrating, can exsanguinate in minutes. While lay people and first responders can do little outside of the hospital to control internal hemorrhage, they can act quickly to control external hemorrhage. The Stop the Bleed program focuses on training to control life-threatening external hemorrhage with the fundamental concept that "no one should die from uncontrolled bleeding." Once the victim has been identified, the closest person to render help may likely not have any medical training. Thus, if the lay person can initiate care, it can buy time until police, fire, and/or emergency medical services arrive to provide additional care and transport the patient to a trauma center for definitive care.

The key principles of Stop the Bleed are to ensure your own safety, call 911, identify the injury, and stop the bleeding. After you ensure your own safety, then it is appropriate to offer help. You might need to direct someone to call 911, or do it yourself. Make every effort to protect yourself from blood-borne pathogens by wearing gloves. Remove the clothing over the victim's wounds to completely expose and evaluate the injury and reveal hidden injuries.

The acronym **THREAT** is used to enact the Stop the Bleed action plan:

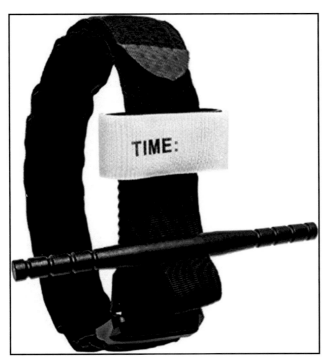

Figure 9-11. Tourniquet.

- Threat suppression
- Hemorrhage control
- Rapid Extrication to safety
- Assessment by medical providers
- Transport to definitive care

The major causes of death from bleeding, excluding internal bleeding in the chest and abdomen, are due to issues in the extremities, neck, shoulders, axilla, and groin regions. Large arteries and veins traverse these regions, and, if untreated, exsanguination can occur quickly.

External Hemorrhage Control

External hemorrhage control is best obtained by applying direct pressure to the wound. If the wound is on the extremities and direct pressure is not effective or practical, or the bleeding is obviously life-threatening, a tourniquet should be applied promptly. If the wound is not amenable to a tourniquet, then wound packing and hemostatic agents should be considered.

Tourniquet

The tourniquet (Figure 9-11) should be applied high and tight on the extremity and tightened until the bleeding stops. If applying the initial tourniquet does not control the bleeding, a second can be applied just above the first. Properly applied tourniquets stop arterial blood flow into the extremity and from the wound. However, despite the tourniquet's proper application, it can cause pain. The tourniquet should not be removed or loosened unless done

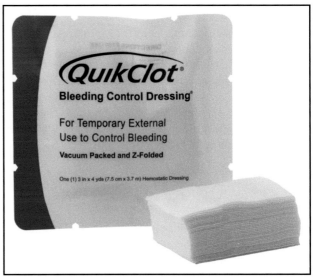

Figure 9-12. Hemostatic agent, QuickClot.

by a physician or under a physician's guidance. Although a makeshift tourniquet such as a belt can be used, a commercially manufactured tourniquet should be available at all athletic venues.

Wound Packing

If direct pressure fails, wound packing should be performed for life-threatening bleeding from the neck, shoulder, axilla, and groin regions. The wound can be packed with either a hemostatic dressing or plain gauze rolls. The packing needs to be placed tightly in the wound and directly onto the source of bleeding. Direct pressure should be held for 3 minutes if using a hemostatic agent and for 10 minutes if using a plain gauze roll. If, after the appropriate period of time, the initial packing fails to control the hemorrhage, a second gauze can be placed on top of the first, followed by the reapplication of direct pressure.

Hemostatic Agents

Hemostatic agents (Figure 9-12) are designed to promote rapid blood coagulation in the event of life-threatening or potentially life-threatening hemorrhage. They can be powder, granules, or impregnated gauze. QuikClot (Z-Medica LLC) was originally available as a powder and was designed to be directly poured on the wound to absorb the water in the blood, thus increasing its clotting capabilities. Zeolite was the second formulation of QuikClot as granules, which created an exothermic reaction. However, it was not available for commercial use and was used only in emergency scenarios such as combat. The hemostatic gauze is impregnated with kaolin, an inorganic mineral that accelerates the body's natural clotting ability without causing an exothermic reaction.

Thermoregulation

All patients with trauma should be kept warm; it's equally as important as controlling hemorrhage. As patients hemorrhage or are exposed to the elements, they become hypothermic, which can lead to coagulopathy and increased bleeding. Often, patients with severe traumatic injury will develop the lethal trauma triad of hypothermia, coagulopathy, and metabolic acidosis, and this results in a significant increase in the mortality rate.

CHAPTER SUMMARY

Patients can sustain penetrating and non-penetrating injuries to the skin, underlying tendons, ligaments, muscle, bones, and organs. The most common injuries are contusions, abrasions, lacerations, burns, and penetrating injuries. All open wounds need to cleansed and treated based on the nature of the injury. Patients with blunt or penetrating injuries can sustain life-threatening internal and external hemorrhages. While little can be done outside of the hospital setting to control internal hemorrhage, Stop the Bleed can be instituted in an effort to control life-threatening external hemorrhage. Tourniquets and wound packing with hemostatic agents can be used safely and effectively to control external hemorrhage.

CHAPTER REVIEW QUESTIONS

1. A 20-year-old male accidentally slips and rolls down a hillside during soccer practice. He crawls up the hillside, bleeding from his right leg, and asks for help. After you lay the player supine, you notice that bright red blood is spurting out of a moderate size wound in the middle of the right thigh. The player is pale and anxious. Which of the following steps would you take to control the bleeding?
   a) place a tourniquet above the right knee
   b) place a tourniquet over the wound
   c) place a tourniquet over the left upper thigh
   d) place a tourniquet over the right upper thigh
   e) place a tourniquet above the left knee

2. A 16-year-old female gets checked with a lacrosse stick during the championship game. She falls and strikes her left upper arm on a large jagged rock. She sustains a laceration approximately 5 cm long and down through the fatty tissue with exposed tendon and bone. Being the team captain, she wants to get "fixed up" and go back into the game. You advise the player that:
   a) you will place butterfly strips over the wound and allow her to return to the game
   b) you will clean out the wound and place a dressing over the area, and she can return to the game
   c) you will clean and suture the wound at halftime, and she can return in the second half
   d) you will clean the wound and place a dressing over the area, and she should not return to play
   e) you have evaluated the wound, and based on the depth and exposed tendon and bone, you will place a dressing over the wound, she will not return to play, and she needs to go to the emergency room for treatment

3. During a football game, a fight breaks out at halftime as the players are returning to the locker room. Once security has control of the situation and the players are in their respective locker rooms, you notice that the 17-year-old lineman is short of breath. He tells you he is fine, does not need anything, and is just winded from the altercation. When he stands up to leave the locker room, he almost passes out from his shortness of breath. The coach asks you to look at him, and you notice a tear in his football jersey on the right side of the chest area. There is some blood on the uniform, but not anything significant. After you call for emergency medical services, your main concern is that the player sustained which of the following injuries?
   a) liver laceration
   b) splenic laceration
   c) superficial wound
   d) pneumothorax
   e) aortic injury

ANSWERS

1. d. Tourniquets should be placed proximal to the injury over the artery. In this case, there is concern for right femoral artery laceration. Thus, the tourniquet should be placed over the right femoral artery on the upper thigh near the groin.

2. e. This player sustained a deep laceration to her right upper extremity that has exposed the tendon and bone. This wound is not amenable to simple wound care, and the player needs to be evaluated for tendon, ligament, and bone injury. The wound requires a thorough washout and closure in the hospital, and may require orthopedic consultation.

3. d. The player sustained a stab wound to the right chest. The most likely injury above the diaphragm is a pneumothorax. Patients will typically present with shortness of breath.

REFERENCES

1. Bryant RA, Nix DP. *Acute and Chronic Wounds: Current Management Concepts*. St. Louis, MO: Elsevier; 2016.

2. Trott AT. *Wounds and Lacerations: Emergency Care and Closure*. Philadelphia, PA: Elsevier/Saunders; 2012.

3. Marx JA, Rosen P. *Rosen's Emergency Medicine: Concepts and Clinical Practice*. Philadelphia, PA: Elsevier/Saunders; 2014.

4. Tintinalli JE, Stapczynski J, Ma OJ, Yealy DM, Meckler GD, Cline DM. *Tintinalli's Emergency Medicine: A Comprehensive Study Guide*. New York: McGraw-Hill Education; 2016.

5. Stop the Bleed Texas EMS Trauma and Acute Care Foundation. June 9. 2019. https://tetaf.org/stop-the-bleed/. Accessed August 26, 2019.

6. Jacobs LM, Wade D, McSwain NF, et al. Hartford consensus: a call to action for THREAT, a medical disaster preparedness concept. *J Am Coll Surg*. 2014;218(3):467-475.

7. Jacobs LM, Mcswain NE, Rotondo MF, et al. Improving survival from active shooter events: the Hartford consensus. *Bull Am Coll Surg*. 2013;98(6):14-16.

8. Jacobs, LM, McSwain, NE, Rotondo, MF, et al. Improving survival from active shooter events: the Hartford consensus. *J Trauma Acute Care Surg*. 2013;74(6):1399-1400.

9. Jacobs, LM. Joint committee to create a national policy to enhance survivability from mass casualty shooting events: the Hartford consensus II. *J Am Coll Surg*. 2014;218(3):476-478.

10. Pons, PT, Jerome, J, McMullen, J. The Hartford consensus on active shooters: implementing the continuum of prehospital trauma response. *J Emerg Med*. 2015;49(6):875-885.

11. Jacobs, LM, Burns, KJ, Langer, G, et. al. The Hartford Consensus: a national survey of the public regarding bleeding control. *J Am Coll Surg*. 2016;222(5):948-955.

10

Epileptic Seizures

Ryan P. McGovern, PhD, LAT, ATC

Chapter Key Words

- Acute care
- Epilepsy
- Nonepileptic seizures
- Sports participation
- Stigma of epilepsy

Chapter Scenario

Shane is the athletic trainer for a Division II collegiate swimming and diving program. After an early-morning practice, he notices a group of student-athletes circled around a teammate. On initial evaluation, the student-athlete is upright and aware. She is an 18-year old freshman who describes an intense feeling that "elevator music was playing on the pool deck" for an unknown amount of time. This happened as she was sitting on the edge of the pool after practice. She reports that she could hear her teammates talking around her, but she could not recall what they were talking about. After her episode, she describes being slightly dazed and confused and tells her teammates to wait with her while she "gets her head straight."

After they arrive at the athletic training room, the student-athlete informs Shane that this is not the first time that something like this has happened. There have been 2 other incidents during her high school career following early-morning workouts. She did not report these to anyone because she thought it was due to the time of occurrence and intensity of the workouts.

How would you classify the type of seizure that this student-athlete experienced? Where would you refer this student-athlete? Could this individual be cleared for return-to-sport, and what special considerations would need to be made for this athlete to continue participation in swimming?

Scenario Resolution

This epileptic seizure would be classified as a focal onset seizure with impaired awareness. Even though the patient was able to mildly interact with her environment, she was not able to interpret her teammates or the circumstances surrounding her, and she demonstrated mild confusion. The athlete should be seen by her primary care physician or team physician, with referral to a specialist with experience in the treatment of epilepsy. This athlete would be considered for a return-to-sport following these referrals and proper management of her condition with antiepileptic drugs and other treatment measures. Special considerations would have to be made during her swimming events. Swimming is a Group 2 sport that does pose some risk to her if an epileptic event were to occur while she was in the water.

Feld F., Gorse KM, Blanc RO
Non-Orthopedic Emergency Care in Athletes (pp 75-00).

INTRODUCTION

Epileptic seizures are defined as a *transient occurrence of signs and/or symptoms due to abnormal, excessive, or synchronous neuronal activities of the brain.*[1] An imbalance in the signaling between neurotransmitters and/or changes in the structural channels within brain cells can cause symptoms that drastically affect a person's quality of life. Changes in the normal electrical brain activity of an individual can result in alterations to awareness, perception, behavior, and/or physical movements.[2] These changes can last from a few seconds to several minutes, depending on the severity of the seizure.

The effects of seizures can cause persistent health-related concerns that have been associated with restrictions in physical activity and sports participation due to fear of causing seizures or increasing the frequency of occurrence.[3,4] Despite medical recommendations encouraging athletic participation for individuals with seizure disorders, studies have demonstrated that those affected are less active and physically fit in comparison to those not affected.[5-8] The stigma around seizures, specifically epilepsy or seizure disorders, has caused individuals to be excluded from sports participation due to "fear, overprotection, and ignorance."[2,5]

When clearing an individual with epilepsy for sports participation, several factors need to be considered, including the type and severity of the seizures, the probability of a seizure occurring and precipitating factors, the usual timing of seizure occurrence, the type of sport participation, and the attitude of the person (and parent/guardian, if warranted) in accepting some level of risk for the athlete's participation.[3] The health care provider for athletes with epilepsy must understand these factors, as well as the risks and benefits of exercise and the current recommendations for the protection and management of individuals with seizure disorders, to promote a positive and safe environment for sports participation.

Epilepsy Epidemiology and Definition

Epilepsy, also known as *seizure disorders*, is the fourth most-common neurological disorder, affecting more than 50 million people, or 2% of the population, worldwide.[4] In the United States alone, more than 3.4 million people (3 million adults and 470,000 children), or 1.2% of the population, report active or current epilepsy.[9] Epilepsy affects people of all ages, races, and ethnicities, especially individuals from the lowest socioeconomical class due to lack of access to a proper management plan.[9] According to the International League Against Epilepsy (ILAE),[10] an individual is diagnosed with epilepsy if he or she meets any of the following conditions:

- Has had at least 2 unprovoked seizures occurring greater than 24 hours apart.

- Has had one unprovoked (or reflex) seizure and a probability of further seizures similar to the general recurrence risk (at least 60%) after 2 unprovoked seizures occurring over the next 10 years.

- Has had a diagnosis of an epilepsy syndrome.

Phases of Epileptic Seizures

While all epileptic seizures have a beginning, middle, and end, the affected individual will not notice or perceive all phases.[11] Common signs and symptoms that can occur throughout the progression of a seizure are shown in Table 10-1.

Prior to the beginning of a seizure, some individuals may experience a prodrome, which involves feelings, sensations, or notable changes in behavior that can precede the seizure by several minutes to several days.[12] The prodrome is not part of the seizure, but it can serve as a warning mechanism to the individual and acute health care provider to take steps to prevent a possible injury.[11]

The beginning stage of a seizure, known as the *aura phase*, is marked by the presence of signs and/or symptoms that are often indescribable by the individual, but can be similar each time a seizure manifests.[11,13] Although an aura can occur before changes in awareness, some people do not experience it, and their seizure begins with a total loss of consciousness.[11]

Epileptic seizures are generally self-limiting and last between 1 and 5 minutes, during which the middle, or *ictal*, phase correlates with the abnormal electrical activity in the brain that defines a seizure event.[11,14] As the ictal phase and seizure end, the individual will enter a postictal state of reorientation.[15,16] This recovery period occurs between the epileptic seizure and the individual's return to a normal baseline. This may take a few minutes or several hours and is often characterized by confusion, drowsiness, headache, and nausea.[15] Following his or her return to a normal baseline, an individual can experience muscle fatigue and exhaustion that can last several days.

Triggers and Triggering Precipitants for Epileptic Seizures

During the prodrome phase, changes can occur due to stimulants or factors known as *triggers*. These are usually identifiable and can be the result of an external stimulant, the individual's mental process, or both.[17] Common examples of external stimulants include eating (eg, hot and spicy food); seeing flashing lights; touching hot water; experiencing visual, vestibular, auditory and/or tangible stimulants; reading; and listening to music.[17]

Changes in cerebral function—including movement, emotion, thoughts, calculations, and cognitive function—can elicit an internal, mental process trigger, as can factors known as *triggering precipitants*.[17] While not stimulants,

TABLE 10-1. COMMON SIGNS AND SYMPTOMS OF A SEIZURE

	AWARENESS, SENSORY, AND EMOTIONAL CHANGES (NON-MOTOR)	PHYSICAL CHANGES (MOTOR)
Before	• Déjà vu • Jamais vu • Smells • Sounds • Tastes • Visual loss or blurring • "Strange" feelings • Fear/panic • Pleasant feelings • Racing thoughts	• Dizzy or lightheaded • Headache • Nausea • Numbness or tingling in extremities
During	• Loss of awareness • Confused, feeling spacey • Periods of forgetfulness or memory lapses • Distracted, daydreaming • Loss of consciousness, unconscious, or "pass out" • Unable to hear • Sounds may be strange or different • Unusual smells (eg, burning rubber) • Unusual tastes • Loss of vision or unable to see • Blurry vision • Flashing lights • Formed visual hallucinations • Numbness, tingling, or electric shock–like feeling in body and extremities • Out-of-body sensations • Feeling detached • Déjà vu • Jamais vu • Body parts feel or look different • Feeling of panic, fear, or impending doom • Pleasant feelings	• Difficulty talking • Unable to swallow with drooling • Repeated blinking of eyes, eyes may move to one side or look upward, or staring • Lack of movement or muscle tone • Tremors, twitching, or jerking movements • Rigid or tense muscles Automatisms of the face or arms or legs • Repeated purposeful movements • Convulsions • Incontinence • Sweating • Pale or flushed skin tone • Dilated pupils • Biting of tongue • Difficulty breathing • Heart palpitations
After	• Slow to respond • Sleepy • Confused • Loss of memory • Difficulty talking or writing • Feeling fuzzy, lightheaded, or dizzy • Feeling depressed, sad, or upset • Scared • Anxious • Frustrated, embarrassed, or ashamed	• Musculoskeletal injuries • Tired or exhausted • Headache • Nausea or upset stomach • Thirsty • General weakness or in one part of the body • Urge to go to the bathroom or incontinence

Adapted from Schachter S, Shafer P, Sirven J. What Happens During A Seizure? Accessed June 10, 2019. ed. https://www.epilepsy.com/learn/about-epilepsy-basics/what-happens-during-seizure. Epilepsy Foundation.

Box 10-1. Energy Drinks

With more than 500 brands of energy drinks available, concern has grown over consumption of these products by adolescents and young adults. These caffeinated or stimulant drinks can cause seizure-like symptoms and, in a small number of individuals, have been shown to cause nonepileptic seizures. It is vital to educate your athletes about limiting energy drink consumption before, during, and after sports participation.

Common Signs and Symptoms: Insomnia, "jittery" or "shaky" feelings, palpitations, headaches, chest pains, and shortness of breath.[19,20]

---

triggering precipitants include stress, sleep deprivation, fatigue, alcohol, drug use, and menstrual cycle, which can all also lead to epileptic seizures.[17,18] When identified, an individual's trigger or triggering precipitant can be limited to increase the effectiveness of a management plan for epileptic seizures.

Classification of Epilepsy Type and Severity

In 2017, the ILAE's Seizure Type Classification Task Force established recommendations for seizure classification.[21] The operational goal of this group was to define seizure types in a way that was easier to interpret in clinical, teaching, and research settings[10] (Figure 10-1). When describing epileptic seizures, 3 main areas of focus are identified for an accurate classification of type: type of onset or beginning of a seizure, the individual's level of awareness throughout the seizure, and whether the individual has movement symptoms during the seizure.[22-24]

Type of onset identifies where the seizure began in the brain and can be classified as focal, generalized, or unknown.[10] A focal-onset seizure originates within networks limited to one side of the brain. It may be discretely localized or more widely distributed. Focal seizures can originate in subcortical or in deep brain structures.[25,26]

Generalized-onset seizures originate at some point within the brain, and rapidly engage in bilaterally distributed networks.[25,26] In other words, a focal-onset seizure affects one hemisphere of the brain, while a generalized-onset seizure affects both.

An unknown-onset seizure is defined when the area of onset is not known or cannot be defined. This distinction is commonly used when the seizure takes place at night or when the individual is alone with no one to witness the event.[10,21,22] As more information is gathered following an unknown seizure, the onset can be redefined to either a focal or generalized onset.[10]

Level of awareness during a seizure is important for practical application, as it can directly affect the individual's safety and the acute health care provider's response to the seizure. For a focal-onset seizure, awareness is defined as either *aware* or *impaired awareness*.[10,21,25] Aware is used if the individual is conscious of him- or herself and the environment during the seizure, while impaired awareness is used if either of these is lost at any point throughout

the seizure.[10] It refers specifically to awareness during the seizure, and not an individual's ability to recall whether a seizure has occurred.[25] During a generalized onset seizure, impaired awareness commonly occurs in most cases and is assumed unless otherwise noted by the witness or acute health care provider.[25] The level of awareness for an unknown-onset seizure cannot be defined due to the absence of a witness during the event.

The identification of motor (physical) or nonmotor (sensory and emotional) symptoms at the start of the seizure is important to the classification type. If both motor and nonmotor symptoms occur at the beginning, motor signs and symptoms will usually dominate.[10] Common motor symptoms include muscles going limp (atonic); muscles twitching (myoclonus); muscles becoming tense or rigid (tonic); rhythmical full-body jerking motions (clonic); and epileptic spasms.[22] Nonmotor symptoms can include sensory or emotional changes as well as changes in the individual's thought process. A comprehensive list of motor and nonmotor symptoms can be found in Table 10-1. Nonmotor symptoms for generalized or unknown onset seizures are also known as *absence seizures*. These often present with a sudden cessation of activity and awareness, as well as staring spells with myoclonus twitching of the eyelids.[22,25] Focal-onset seizures can be further defined as seizures changing from a focal beginning to a bilateral (generalized) tonic–clonic seizure due to the regularity of their occurrence among individuals with epilepsy.[25]

The affected individual commonly assesses the severity of seizures subjectively after all signs and symptoms have subsided to evaluate his or her perception of the physical and emotional response to the seizure.[27] The evaluation of severity in individuals with epilepsy is common and is assessed through the use of instruments, including the Seizure Frequency Scoring System, the Veterans Administration Seizure Frequency and Severity Rating Scale, the National Hospital (Chalfont) Seizure Severity Scale, the Occupational Hazard Scale, the Liverpool Seizure Severity Scale, and the Hague Seizure Severity Scale.[27] These scales take into account seizure type, duration of event, frequency of the seizures, physical symptoms during the ictal phase, and duration of the postictal recovery period.[27] While there is not a universal tool for evaluation of seizure severity, acute health care providers for athletes

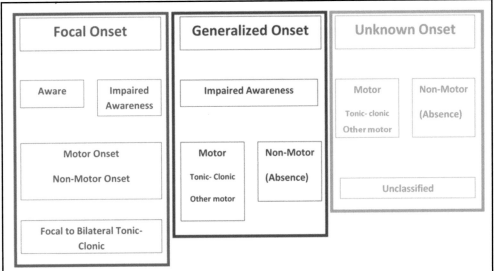

Figure 10-1. International League Against Epilepsy Classification of Seizure Types (Basic Version). (Adapted from Fisher, RS, Cross JH, French JA, et al. Operational classification of seizure types by the International League Against Epilepsy: Position Paper of the ILAE Commission for Classification and Terminology. *Epilepsia.* 2017; 58(4): 522-530.)

with epilepsy should maintain at least one instrument to uniformly track the severity of the seizures.

Epilepsy Diagnosis

Following the first occurrence of a seizure, the individual should be referred to a primary care physician and a specialist trained in the treatment of epilepsy.[23,24,28] The diagnosis of epilepsy or epilepsy syndrome is largely predicated on a comprehensive clinical evaluation, with a thorough medical history from both the affected individual and witnesses to the seizure or seizure events. The clinical history can vary but should include circumstances under which the seizure occurred, timing of the seizure, whether the individual was awake or asleep, whether the individual was standing or sitting, any activity or exercise the individual was doing, possible triggers, precipitating factors, and personal and/or family medical history.[23,24,29] A physical examination should also be performed to address cardiac, neurological, and mental status, and it should include a developmental assessment when deemed appropriate by the specialist.[23,24]

While most cases can be diagnosed through a comprehensive medical history and physical exam, some need video recordings of the event and electroencephalography testing to document visible signs and symptoms, as well as abnormalities in the electrical activity of the brain.[23,29,30] A comprehensive evaluation is necessary to identify whether individuals are experiencing epileptic seizures and, if so, to diagnose them for specific type of epilepsy.

Epilepsy syndrome is a composite of signs and symptoms that define a unique epilepsy condition.[29] Clinically, this is performed by analyzing the individual's type of epilepsy, age of onset, and associated comorbidities.[31] The defining of specific epilepsy syndromes is commonly associated with clinical findings and electroencephalography testing. Examples of epilepsy syndromes include childhood absence epilepsy, juvenile absence epilepsy, juvenile myoclonic epilepsy, West syndrome, epilepsy with generalized tonic–clonic seizures, idiopathic generalized epilepsy, Panayiotopoulos syndrome, late-onset childhood occipital syndrome, Dravet syndrome, Lennox-Gastaut syndrome, and Landau-Kleffner syndrome.[23,31] Epilepsy syndromes are considered to be resolved for individuals who had an age-dependent epilepsy syndrome but are now past the applicable age for that specific syndrome, as well as those who have remained seizure-free for the past 10 years and without the use of seizure medicines for the past 5 years.[1]

While most individuals are diagnosed with epilepsy following large dramatic events, the minor episodes attributed to lesser signs and symptoms often go overlooked. The accurate understanding and identification of minor seizure events could be critical to making an accurate diagnosis of epilepsy.[24] Acute health care providers must be cognizant of the identification of signs and symptoms of seizures, regardless of how small or insignificant they might be to the affected individual.

Epilepsy Treatment

The goal for treatment of epileptic seizures should be to control or stop the seizures, as well as their side effects.[32] While seizures may be difficult to control, it is imperative that each individual has a treatment plan personally tailored to his or her needs. Treatment plans should only be initiated by a specialist trained in the treatment of epilepsy, along with the individual's primary care physician.[24,28] Most treatment plans will incorporate several aspects that can include antiepileptic drugs, psychological interventions, dietary therapy, neuromodulation, and surgery. The acute health care provider must ensure that each individual has an identified treatment plan to control or stop epileptic seizures, as prescribed by a specialist in the treatment of epilepsy.

TABLE 10-2. COMMONLY PRESCRIBED ANTIEPILEPTIC DRUGS

• Carbamazepine	• Oxcarbazepine
• Clobazam	• Phenobarbital
• Clonazepam	• Phenytoin
• Eslicarbazepine acetate	• Pregabalin
• Ethosuximide	• Sodium valproate
• Gabapentin	• Tiagabine
• Lacosamide	• Topiramate
• Lamotrigine	• Vigabatrin
• Levetiracetam	• Zonisamide

Adapted from Nunes VD, Sawyer L, Neilson J, Sarri G, Cross JH. Diagnosis and management of the epilepsies in adults and children: summary of updated NICE guidance. *BMJ*. 2012;344:e281

BOX 10-2. ATTENTION-DEFICIT/HYPERACTIVITY DISORDER

Medication has become the mainstay treatment for individuals diagnosed with attention-deficit/hyperactivity disorder. If stimulants are used for treatment, side effects that mimic seizure-like signs and symptoms can occur. Keep up-to-date medication information on all your athletes!

Common Signs and Symptoms: Insomnia, headaches, and increased heart rate and blood pressure.[38,39]

Antiepileptic drugs, prescribed to prevent the recurrence of seizures, form the standard treatment of care for individuals with epilepsy.[23,24] About 65% to 70% of adults and adolescents with epileptic seizures can be successfully controlled with the initially prescribed antiepileptic drug, while an additional 15% to 20% will attain effective control with subsequent antiepileptic drug prescriptions.[32,33] The choice of specific antiepileptic drugs is affected by the classification of seizure type, the individual's age, comorbidities, comedications, lifestyle, possible pregnancy, type of epilepsy syndrome, and preferences of the person and family members as appropriate.[23,24,28] Antiepileptic drugs make up a diverse group of medications with different properties and mechanisms of action that contribute to their therapeutic effects.[34,35] While it is beyond the scope of this publication to differentiate between them, commonly prescribed antiepileptic drugs are listed in Table 10-2.

It is recommended that antiepileptic drugs be chosen on the basis of the epilepsy syndrome, or, if not clear at presentation, then on the type of epileptic seizure.[23,24] The acute health care provider for athletes with epilepsy should be diligent in identifying any possible adverse effects or changes in behavior of their athletes while they are on prescribed antiepileptic drugs.[23] While antiepileptic drugs have been successful in treating individuals with epilepsy, 25% to 35% of individuals will not be able to control their seizures with medication.[36,37] Other therapies should be considered if the epilepsy is not controlled with only medication within 2 years, management has been unsuccessful

following administration of 2 antiepileptic drugs, the individual is experiencing adverse side effects from the medication, a psychological and/or psychiatric comorbidity has been diagnosed; or diagnostic doubt exists regarding the type of epilepsy or epilepsy syndrome.

Psychological interventions should be considered for use in conjunction with antiepileptic drugs, but not as an alternative to the medication.[24] Cognitive dysfunction and psychiatric comorbidities have been shown to be more prevalent in individuals with epilepsy than among the general population.[40-42] If left untreated, psychological and psychiatric conditions have a greater negative effect on the individual's quality of life than the seizure-related signs and symptoms.[40,41,43] Relaxation techniques, cognitive behavior therapy, and biofeedback have been shown to improve the quality of life for some individuals, but have not been proven to decrease the frequency of seizures. In adolescents, specific attention should be shown to their relationships with friends, teammates, and families.[24] Acute health care providers are commonly the first line of defense in reporting changes in behavior among their athletes.

Dietary therapy has been shown to be effective in the treatment of some individuals with refractory, or uncontrolled, seizures, usually along with antiepileptic drug administration. Specifically, the ketogenic diet has shown an ability to maintain the presence of ketone bodies (compounds produced during the metabolism of fats) in circulation, which have an antiepileptic effect, although the exact mechanism is not clearly defined.[31,36] This specialized

> ## Box 10-3. Cannabidiol Oil
>
> Cannabidiol oil is a constituent of the cannabis plant that does not elicit euphoria and may significantly decrease the frequency of seizures in individuals with epilepsy. While it is not considered a widely used therapy, it is a topic that needs to be monitored by acute health care providers for athletes with epilepsy.[46-48]

diet contains a 4:1 ratio of fats to carbohydrates, with the amount of protein regulated so that about 90% of calories are derived from consumption of fats.[36] This diet should be prescribed and monitored by a specialist in epilepsy, along with a nutritionist. While this approach has demonstrated clinically meaningful improvements, compliance with administration of this highly unusual diet can be challenging.[31,36,37] The modified Atkins diet is a high-fat, low-carbohydrate option that has had similar effects to the ketogenic diet, but it is far less restrictive, which can make it easier for an athlete to maintain compliance.[37] While long-term adherence to both diets can be challenging, especially in athletes, the effects can be felt in a short amount of time and have been shown to be successful in individuals with refractory seizures.[31,37]

The most commonly used form of neuromodulation in individuals with epilepsy is through stimulation of the vagus nerve. This treatment is indicated for use when antiepileptic drugs have not been successful in reducing the frequency of epileptic seizures.[24] This should be considered an adjunctive therapy used with the continued administration of antiepileptic drugs. A battery-powered apparatus is implanted into the individual's chest, like a pacemaker, with a wire extending to the left vagus nerve in the neck.[24] The treatment regimen for application of pulses through the device will vary by individual. Special considerations and medical clearances should be made for individuals who wish to participate in athletic activity or sports under the supervision of the primary care provider and specialist in the treatment of epilepsy.

For individuals who have not had success with antiepileptic drug administration and other treatment options, surgical intervention may be warranted. Positive long-term outcomes have been reported in significantly reducing seizure frequency with certain types of surgical interventions.[44] Psychosocial outcomes have also been shown to improve an individual's quality of life following surgical intervention.[45] Surgery is considered only after every other treatment course has been fully exhausted, with no change to the frequency, severity, and side effects of the seizures.

Epilepsy Management

A comprehensive management plan must be established and agreed upon by all parties involved, including the affected individual, his or her family, the primary care provider, and a specialist in the treatment of epilepsy.[23,24] It is the role of the acute health care provider to ensure that each individual has an identified management plan to control epileptic seizures prior to consideration, medical clearance, and participation in a sports activity.

Epilepsy and Sports Participation

History

In 1968, the American Medical Association Committee on the Medical Aspects of Sports and the Committee on Exercise and Physical Fitness first endorsed the concept that individuals with seizure disorders were safe to participate in sports activities.[5,49] Participation was encouraged, provided that the individual's seizures were under control and that the type of athletic activity would not increase the frequency of seizures or expose the athlete to repeated head trauma.[49] Following a research article published in 1973, the American Medical Association acknowledged that individuals could participate in any sport, including contact and collision sports, provided that all safeguards were taken to prevent head injuries.[5,50,51] Each case of participation was to be evaluated individually, with the emphasis put on noncontact sports if possible, barring any psychosocial factors that necessitated participation in contact sports.[5,52]

In 1983, the American Academy of Pediatrics Committee on Children With Handicaps and the Committee on Sports Medicine released the first position statement recommending that sports participation for adolescents and young adults with epilepsy and seizure disorders was safe and beneficial from a health and psychosocial standpoint.[5,53] Since then, the ILAE Task Force on Sports and Epilepsy has published 2 international position statements on sports participation by those with epilepsy, first in 1997 and most recently in 2016.[3,54] The purpose of these statements has been to guide the safe participation of individuals with epilepsy in exercise and sports, and to suggest recommendations for the issuance of medical certificates for participation in sports activities.[3] A thorough preparticipation evaluation should be performed prior to sports participation and at each subsequent sports season to ensure that seizure type and frequency have not changed, as well as to establish any seizure-related injuries, duration of symptoms and seizure-free timeframes, and adherence to antiepileptic drugs and/or other treatments.[3,51,55] In 2014, the National Athletic Training Association recommended that all athletes with a seizure disorder should undergo a thorough neurological screening as part of their preparticipation evaluation.[56]

Individuals with epilepsy have commonly been advised to avoid exercise and sports activities due to the irregular pathology of epilepsy as well as the fear of causing seizures, increasing the frequency of seizures, and/or sustaining injuries due to uncontrolled seizures.[3,4] However, the available research states that physical activity and active participation in sports can positively affect seizure control as well as improve the overall physical and psychosocial quality of life for the individual with epilepsy.[3] To promote a positive and safe environment for sports participation, the health care provider for athletes with epilepsy needs to understand the risks and benefits of exercise and sports participation, classification of sports based on risk, and the current recommendations for the protection and management of individuals with epilepsy.

Risks and Benefits of Sports Participation

When determining whether an individual with epilepsy can participate in a specific sport, a thorough clinical assessment of the individual's risk-to-benefit ratio must be performed.[3] This analysis should be dependent on the type of seizure and the likelihood of a seizure event occurring during sports participation. The risk of seizures and associated injuries is elevated in individuals with uncontrolled epilepsy, high seizure frequency, and those with comorbidities and mental retardation. The type of seizure is important when making clearances for sports participation, as some types will place the individual in a higher risk category for injury, specifically among those with tonic–clonic seizures that can induce unexpected unconsciousness and unprotected falls. Recommendations that should also be considered before clearing an individual for participation in a specific sport include precipitating factors and the consistency of prodromal indicators, the type of sport participation, and the attitude of the person (and parent or guardian, if warranted) in accepting some level of risk for participation.[3] The primary concern regarding epilepsy and physical activity is the initiation of seizures and secondary injuries that can occur during sports participation.

Theoretically, in relation to exercise and sports activities, risk factors associated with epileptic seizures include fatigue, physical and psychological stress, hyperventilation, excessive aerobic exercise, and metabolic changes due to antiepileptic drug usage.[3,51,55,57,58] However, epileptic seizures have rarely been triggered by participation in physical exercise or sports activity.

There has been no established link between exercise or sports participation and an increase in seizure frequency due to post-activity fatigue. Physical stress has been identified as a seizure trigger for a large number of individuals with epilepsy[51,55,57,59]; however, the same stress elicited during exercise might also activate hormones that could decrease the individual's susceptibility to seizures.[4,5,51] Hyperventilation can be attributed to increased aerobic activity during certain exercise or sports participation. While hyperventilation at rest has been shown to increase confusion and decrease awareness in individuals with epilepsy, the physiological response to an increase in metabolic demand during exercise may actually cause a suppression of abnormalities observed between seizure events.[4,51,57] Excessive aerobic activity has been reported to increase the frequency of these seizures, yet due to its recognized association, individuals will avoid this activity by participating in different sports.[51,57] Other studies have demonstrated that an increase in aerobic exercise will decrease the frequency of seizures due to the psychological benefit of the individual's mental activation to suppress epileptic triggers.

Overall, aerobic exercise, with its general health and psychological benefits, is recommended for individuals with epilepsy, despite the fact that it may trigger seizures in certain populations.[58] The increase in the individual's metabolic demand attained during exercise has been thought to increase the metabolism of antiepileptic drug absorption, causing an increase in the amount of medication in the blood.[51,57] However, there is conflicting evidence, and it is recommended that serum levels should be evaluated only if indicated clinically by the treating primary care physician and specialist in the treatment of epilepsy.

The susceptibility to physical injuries associated with sports participation is frequently the primary reason why individuals with epilepsy have been restricted from activity. The fear of injury due to a sudden fall without warning during sports participation has contributed to low levels of physical activity in individuals with epilepsy.[4] Commonly discussed is the occurrence of minor head injuries caused by epileptic seizures during sports participation.[51] As a whole, there is no evidence that demonstrates that repetitive minor head trauma will increase the frequency or severity of epileptic seizures. This has specifically been shown in individuals participating in contact and collision sports such as football, hockey, and soccer.[5,60] Individuals with controlled epilepsy should not be restricted from participating in contact and collision sports; however, normal safety precautions should be used.[58] The most common injuries sustained by individuals with epilepsy are soft-tissue injuries, but these frequently occur at home, not during sports participation.[51,61] Despite the lack of evidence demonstrating injuries sustained during sports, individuals with epilepsy participate at a lower rate than their healthy counterparts.

The available evidence suggests that exercise can improve the signs, symptoms, and comorbidities often associated with epilepsy. Physical activity can decrease seizure frequency and severity as well as lead to improved cardiovascular and psychological health in people with epilepsy.[5,59] Exercise has a positive effect on maximal aerobic capacity, work capacity, weight and body fat reduction, and decreased risk factors related to conditions associated with a sedentary lifestyle.[2,5,59,62] Improvements to an epileptic individual's quality of life through sports participation

TABLE 10-3. CATEGORIZATION OF SPORTS BY RISK OF INJURY OR DEATH

GROUP 1 (NO SIGNIFICANT RISK)	GROUP 2 (MODERATE RISK BUT NOT FOR BYSTANDERS)	GROUP 3 (HIGH RISK AND FOR BYSTANDERS)

• Athletics
  ◦ except for sports in group 2
• Baseball
• Basketball
• Bowling
• Cricket
• Cross-country skiing
• Curling
• Dancing
• Field hockey
• Football
• Golf
• Judo
• Racquet sports
  ◦ squash, table tennis, tennis
• Rugby
• Volleyball
• Wrestling
	• Alpine skiing
	• Archery
	• Athletics
	  ◦ pole vault
	• Biathlon, triathlon, pentathlon
	• Boxing
	• Canoeing
	• Cycling
	• Fencing
	• Gymnastics
	• Horse riding
	• Ice hockey
	• Karate
	• Shooting
	• Skateboarding
	• Skating
	• Snowboarding
	• Swimming
	• Water skiing
	• Weightlifting
		• Aviation
		• Climbing
		• Diving
		• Horse racing (competitive)
		• Motor sports
		• Parachuting (similar sports)
		• Rodeo
		• Scuba diving
		• Ski jumping
		• Solitary sailing
		• Surfing, windsurfing

Adapted from Capovilla G, Kaufman KR, Perucca E, Moshe SL, Arida RM. Epilepsy, seizures, physical exercise, and sports: A report from the ILAE Task Force on Sports and Epilepsy. *Epilepsia*. 2016;57(1):6-12.

could lower levels of depression, improve mood, and enhance self-esteem.[2,51,63]

Recent studies have begun evaluating the overall effect of exercise on the cognitive function of individuals with epilepsy.[64] While such research is still in its infancy, there is hope that an increase in physical activity and exercise can be shown to have the same positive effects on cognition that it has in the normal population.[64,65] Exercise and sports participation should be encouraged by the acute health care provider on an individual basis as long as the benefits outweigh the risks.

Classification of Sports

The primary care physician and a specialist treating the epileptic individual should conduct a systematic pre-participation physical examination to safely clear the athlete for sports participation. This should be performed to determine whether participation in a particular sport is safe for the affected individual, the acute health care provider, and the sport bystanders.[3] Sports have been classified on the basis of potential risk of injury to the individual and

bystanders such as other athletes, referees, and spectators, should an epileptic seizure occur.[3] These sports have been assembled into Groups 1 through 3 (Table 10-3). Group 1 sports pose no significant additional risk of injury to epileptic individuals or bystanders. Group 2 sports involve a moderate risk of physical injury to the individual with epilepsy, but not bystanders. Group 3 sports involve a major risk of injury or death to the individual with epilepsy, and, in some sports, also involve risk for bystanders.[3]

Special precautions are not considered necessary for individuals with controlled epilepsy, while those individuals with uncontrolled epilepsy should be assessed individually for contact and collision sports.[51] The only sports that have been consistently contraindicated for individuals with epilepsy involve airborne or free-falling activities such has skydiving, due to the disastrous consequences if a seizure event were to occur in the air.[3,5]

Any final recommendations for participation should be based on the specific circumstances relating to participation, as well as on the judgment of the primary care physician and/or specialist treating the individual with epilepsy.[3] It is also important to distinguish those who are exercising or playing sports in a recreational setting from those who wish to play academically or professionally. The valuation and the intensity of eventual seizure-precipitating factors involved in both situations can vary, and must be taken into account when providing counseling and care for the athlete.[51] The decision to participate in a specific sports activity is ultimately the individual's choice, and because no guidelines are available according to each particular frequency or type of seizure,[3] precautions need to be taken by the acute health care provider during sports participation.

Recommendations for the Acute Health Care Provider

An established management plan is the most effective defense for an emergency seizure event involving an individual with epilepsy during sports participation. The comprehensive plan must be established and agreed upon by all parties involved, including the affected individual, the person's family, the primary care physician and specialist in the treatment of epilepsy, and the acute care management team including the athletic trainer and team physician.[23,24] The acute health care provider for epileptic athletes must ensure that each individual has an established plan to control epileptic seizures prior to consideration of participation, medical clearance, and involvement in sports activities. The continued participation of the individual is based on his or her ability to maintain and communicate the sustained use of this management plan. All standard safety precautions should be used when acutely caring for an athlete, including athletic supervision and the use of appropriate protective equipment in sports that require such measures.[2,5] An amendment to the emergency action plan for each sports facility and location should include a protocol for emergencies involving a seizure event (Appendix 4).

A rapid emergency response plan is necessary for the acute care management of an individual following a seizure event. Acute health care providers should first follow the basic rules of first aid by checking the scene; evaluating the athlete for airway, breathing, and circulation; and providing any necessary life-saving measures.[24,66] Maintenance of a safe environment surrounding the athlete is essential throughout the seizure, especially if the athlete is experiencing uncontrolled motor changes such as during a tonic–clonic seizure. This can require the acute health care provider to help the athlete to the ground or to a safer location, as well as supporting the individual's head to prevent uncontrolled contact with the floor.[66,67] A seizing individual should never be restrained, nor should anything be placed in the mouth unless necessary for life-saving procedures following the seizure event.[66,67] A seizure normally lasts between 1 and 5 minutes, so prevention of self-injury should be the acute health care provider's primary responsibility.[66] When the athlete is entering the postictal state, he or she should be positioned on the side in a recovery position to avoid aspiration.[66] Emergency medical services should be activated if:

1. it is the individual's first experience with a seizure;
2. the seizure lasts longer than 5 minutes or longer than a prior seizure event;
3. the individual remains in an unconscious state; or
4. there are concerns or difficulties maintaining the person's airway, breathing, and circulation and/or other vital signs.[24,66]

The clinical diagnosis and management of epileptic seizures are largely predicated on a thorough history from both the affected individual and witnesses to the seizure. As the primary witness, the acute health care provider should record everything that occurred before, during, and after the seizure event.[68] A sample observation form is provided in Figure 10-2 to help guide the recording of such events.[68] Particular attention should be paid to elements of consciousness throughout the entire seizure; awareness of ongoing activities around the athlete; the time frame encompassing the event (eg, aura phase, onset, duration, ending, and postictal phase); responsiveness of the individual to verbal or nonverbal stimuli; and the overall sense of self as being distinct from others.[25] The ability of the acute health care provider to maintain a calm demeanor throughout the seizure will enable a more accurate recollection of events. This should be founded in the preparation and maintenance of an effective emergency action plan for seizure emergencies.[66]

Status epilepticus (SE), an acute medical emergency that can arise from an epileptic seizure, is associated with significant morbidity and mortality among children.[69,70] SE is defined as seizure activity lasting more than 30 minutes or the occurrence of 2 or more seizures without regaining consciousness.[69,70] For the acute health care provider, a seizure lasting longer than 5 minutes or significantly longer than the normal occurrence for an individual with epilepsy should be considered as SE.[70] Quick treatment with one or several rescue medications is necessary to prevent long-term effects.[71] The management plan for the acute medical emergency of SE should be prescribed by the individual's primary care physician and/or specialist in the treatment of epilepsy.[72] Medications are most effectively administered intravenously; however, for the acute care provider, alternate routes of administration can involve rectal, buccal, intrapulmonary, subcutaneous, intramuscular, and intranasal treatments.[71] These should only be administered by trained clinical personnel or acute health care providers with appropriate training, if specified by an agreed protocol drawn up with the individual's primary care physician and/or specialist in the treatment of epilepsy. The activation of emergency medical services should be performed immediately in situations of SE, even with the administration of preapproved rescue medication.

1. Behavior BEFORE Seizure

Athletic or Sporting Event (location/practice or game/environmental conditions/other):

Change in Behavior: YES/NO

Possible Triggers or Precipitating Factors:

2. Signs and Symptoms DURING Seizure

Changes in Awareness:

Ability to Speak: YES/NO

Responsiveness to Verbal Commands: YES/NO

Incontinence: YES/NO

Physical Symptoms (movements, repeated movements, muscle tone, skin color, sweating, heavy breathing): *Specify where the symptoms began and spread, including extremity (left/right/both)*

3. Behavior AFTER Seizure

Response to Verbal Commands or Physical Touch:

Ability to Communicate (verbally or physically):

Awareness of Name, Place, Time, and Who the Observer is:

Emotional Response and Mood:

Weakness/Numbness/Inability to Regain Any Normal Function:

Tired/Sleepiness: YES/NO

Additional Comments:

Figure 10-2. Seizure observation form. (Adapted from Schachter S, Shafer P, and Sirven J. Seizure Response Plan 101. October 23, 2013 ed. https://www.epilepsy.com/learn/managing-your-epilepsy/seizure-response-plans-101: Epilepsy Foundation. Accessed June 11, 2019.)

Stigma of Epilepsy and Sports Participation

Due to the stigma often associated with epilepsy, individuals with epilepsy are more likely to have lower self-esteem, fewer close relationships, and higher suicide rates.[55] Physical activity has been shown to decrease seizure frequency and severity, as well as lead to improved cardiovascular and psychological health.[5,59] Despite this, individuals commonly avoid sports participation or hide their diagnosis from teammates due to the fear of being viewed differently because of the lack of understanding among the general population.[73] Acceptance of individuals with epilepsy in the sports community could help lower levels of depression and improve the social interaction and overall self-esteem of those affected.[2,51,63,73] The sports medicine community has a responsibility to educate others in an effort to improve the quality of life of its epileptic athletes and decrease the stigma associated with epilepsy.[24,51]

Communication among the acute health care providers and coaches can improve the acceptance of epileptic individuals within the sports community, especially those participating in team-oriented sports.

Nonepileptic Seizures

When managing an individual's first occurrence with a seizure event, the acute health care provider must be aware of differential diagnoses commonly associated with epilepsy. Signs and symptoms that mimic an epileptic seizure event can be caused by conditions that include fainting (syncope), mini-strokes (transient ischemic attacks), low blood sugar (hypoglycemia), migraine with confusion, vertigo, sleep disorders (narcolepsy), movement disorders (tics, tremors, and dystonia), metabolic disorders, panic attacks, cardiac disorders, hyponatremia (especially in endurance athletes), trauma associated with a severe head injury, and psychogenic nonepileptic seizures (due to psychological disturbances).[23,24,29]

Due to the difficulty of diagnosing epilepsy, all athletes who experience seizure-like signs and symptoms should be evaluated by their primary care physician and, if deemed necessary, a specialist in the treatment of epilepsy to rule out any differential diagnoses and identify the underlying pathology of the seizure event. The emergency action plan for seizure-like signs and symptoms and nonepileptic seizures should follow the same emergency management plan for epileptic seizures. Convulsions or seizure-like symptoms due to a severe head injury sustained during sports participation should be treated with the established emergency action plan for a traumatic head injury and/or spinal injury.

CHAPTER SUMMARY

The effects of seizures can cause persistent health-related concerns that have been associated with restrictions in physical activity and sports participation due to fear of causing seizures, increasing the frequency of occurrence, or sustaining injuries due to uncontrolled seizures. Despite medical recommendations encouraging athletic participation for individuals with seizure disorders, studies have demonstrated that those affected are less active and less physically fit compared to those not affected. The acute health care provider should encourage exercise and sports participation on an individual basis as long as the benefits outweigh the risks.

It is the role of the acute health care provider for athletes with epilepsy to ensure that each individual has an identified management plan to control epileptic seizures prior to consideration, medical clearance, and participation in a specific sports activity. The comprehensive management plan must be established and agreed upon by all parties involved, including the affected individual, his or her family, the primary care physician and specialist in the treatment of epilepsy, and the acute care management team. A thorough evaluation should be performed prior to sports participation and each subsequent sports season to ensure that seizure type and frequency have not changed, as well as to establish any seizure-related injuries, duration of symptoms and seizure-free time frames, and adherence of the individual to antiepileptic drugs and/or other treatments.

The sports medicine community has a responsibility to educate others in an effort to improve the epileptic athlete's quality of life and decrease the stigma associated with epilepsy. Communication among the acute health care providers and coaches can improve the sports community's acceptance of epileptic individuals, especially those participating in team-oriented sports.

CHAPTER REVIEW QUESTIONS

1. Define epilepsy.
2. What is the most important component of the comprehensive clinical exam in diagnosing an individual with epilepsy?
3. What are the 3 phases that make up a seizure? Name 2 common signs and symptoms for each phase.
4. Define the 3 main areas of focus used to identify the classification of seizure type.
5. Name 5 commonly reported triggers or precipitating factors.

ANSWERS

1. According to the International League Against Epilepsy,[10] an individual is diagnosed with epilepsy if he or she meets any of the following conditions:
   - Has had at least 2 unprovoked seizures occurring greater than 24 hours apart.
   - Has had one unprovoked (or reflex) seizure and a probability of further seizures similar to the general recurrence risk (at least 60%) after 2 unprovoked seizures, occurring over the next 10 years.
   - Has had a diagnosis of an epilepsy syndrome.

2. The diagnosis of epilepsy or epilepsy syndrome is largely predicated on a comprehensive clinical evaluation, with a thorough medical history from both the affected individual and witnesses to the seizure or seizure events.

3. Aura phase, ictal phase, and postictal phase. Common signs and symptoms are listed in Table 10-1.

4. When describing epileptic seizures, the following 3 main areas of focus are identified for an accurate classification of type: type of onset or beginning of a seizure, an individual's level of awareness throughout the seizure, and whether the individual has movement symptoms during the seizure.

5. Common examples of external stimulants include eating (eg, hot and spicy food); seeing flashing lights; touching hot water; experiencing visual, vestibular, auditory and/or tangible stimulants; reading; and listening to music.[17] While not stimulants, triggering precipitants include stress, sleep deprivation, fatigue, alcohol, drug use, and menstrual cycle, which can also all lead to epileptic seizures.[17,18]

REFERENCES

1. Fisher RS, van Emde Boas W, Blume W, et al. Epileptic seizures and epilepsy: definitions proposed by the International League Against Epilepsy (ILAE) and the International Bureau for Epilepsy (IBE). *Epilepsia*. 2005;46(4):470-472.
2. Manuel C, Feinstein R. Sports participation for young athletes with medical conditions: Seizure disorder, infections and single organs. *Curr Probl Pediatr Adolesc Health Care*. 2018;48(5-6):161-171.
3. Capovilla G, Kaufman KR, Perucca E, Moshe SL, Arida RM. Epilepsy, seizures, physical exercise, and sports: a report from the ILAE task force on sports and epilepsy. *Epilepsia*. 2016;57(1):6-12.
4. Arida RM, Cavalheiro EA, da Silva AC, Scorza FA. Physical activity and epilepsy: proven and predicted benefits. *Sports Med*. 2008;38(7):607-615.
5. Knowles BD, Pleacher MD. Athletes with seizure disorders. *Curr Sports Med Rep*. 2012;11(1):16-20.
6. Steinhoff BJ, Neususs K, Thegeder H, Reimers CD. Leisure time activity and physical fitness in patients with epilepsy. *Epilepsia*. 1996;37(12):1221-1227.
7. Bjorholt PG, Nakken KO, Rohme K, Hansen H. Leisure time habits and physical fitness in adults with epilepsy. *Epilepsia*. 1990;31(1):83-87.
8. Jalava M, Sillanpaa M. Physical activity, health-related fitness, and health experience in adults with childhood-onset epilepsy: a controlled study. *Epilepsia*. 1997;38(4):424-429.
9. Zack MM, Kobau R. National and state estimates of the numbers of adults and children with active epilepsy - United States, 2015. *MMWR Morb Mortal Wkly Rep*. 2017;66(31):821-825.
10. Fisher RS, Cross JH, French JA, et al. Operational classification of seizure types by the International League Against Epilepsy: position paper of the ILAE commission for classification and terminology. *Epilepsia*. 2017;58(4):522-530.
11. Epilepsy Foundation. What Happens During a Seizure? https://www.epilepsy.com/learn/about-epilepsy-basics/what-happens-during-seizure. Accessed September 7, 2018.
12. Besag FMC, Vasey MJ. Prodrome in epilepsy. *Epilepsy Behav*. 2018;83:219-233.
13. Seshia SS, McLachlan RS. Aura continua. *Epilepsia*. 2005;46(3):454-455.
14. Mula M. Epilepsy-induced behavioral changes during the ictal phase. *Epilepsy Behav*. 2014;30:14-16.
15. Fisher RS, Engel JJ Jr. Definition of the postictal state: when does it start and end? *Epilepsy Behav*. 2010;19(2):100-104.
16. Harrast MA, Finnoff JT. *Sports Medicine: Study Guide and Review for Boards*. New York, NY: Demos Medical Publishing; 2012. Springer Publishing Company; 2011.
17. Okudan ZV, Ozkara C. Reflex epilepsy: triggers and management strategies. *Neuropsychiatr Dis Treat*. 2018;14:327-337.
18. Ferlisi M, Shorvon S. Seizure precipitants (triggering factors) in patients with epilepsy. *Epilepsy Behav*. 2014;33:101-105.
19. Nordt SP, Vilke GM, Clark RF, et al. Energy drink use and adverse effects among emergency department patients. *J Community Health*. 2012;37(5):976-981.
20. Nordt SP, Claudius I, Rangan C, et al. Reasons for energy drink use and reported adverse effects among adolescent emergency department patients. *Pediatr Emerg Care*. 2017;33(12):770-773.
21. Fisher RS. The new classification of seizures by the International League Against Epilepsy 2017. *Curr Neurol Neurosci Rep*. 2017;17(6):48.
22. Epilepsy Foundation. Types of Seizures. https://www.epilepsy.com/learn/types-seizures. Accessed September 11, 2018.
23. Nunes VD, Sawyer L, Neilson J, Sarri G, Cross JH. Diagnosis and management of the epilepsies in adults and children: summary of updated NICE guidance. *BMJ*. 2012;344:e281.
24. National Clinical Guideline C. National Institute for Health and Clinical Excellence: Guidance. *The Epilepsies: The Diagnosis and Management of the Epilepsies in Adults and Children in Primary and Secondary Care: Pharmacological Update of Clinical Guideline 20*. London: Royal College of Physicians (UK) National Clinical Guideline Centre; 2012.
25. Fisher RS, Cross JH, D'Souza C, et al. Instruction manual for the ILAE 2017 operational classification of seizure types. *Epilepsia*. 2017;58(4):531-542.
26. Berg AT, Millichap JJ. The 2010 revised classification of seizures and epilepsy. *Continuum (Minneap Minn)*. 2013;19(3 Epilepsy):571-597.
27. Thurman DJ, Beghi E, Begley CE, et al. Standards for epidemiologic studies and surveillance of epilepsy. *Epilepsia*. 2011;52 Suppl 7:2-26.
28. Anderson J, Moor CC. Anti-epileptic drugs: a guide for the non-neurologist. *Clin Med (Lond)*. 2010;10(1):54-58.
29. Panayiotopoulos CP. *The Epilepsies: Seizures, Syndromes and Management*. Oxfordshire (UK): Bladon Medical Publishing; 2005.

30. Lawley A, Evans S, Manfredonia F, Cavanna AE. The role of outpatient ambulatory electroencephalography in the diagnosis and management of adults with epilepsy or nonepileptic attack disorder: A systematic literature review. *Epilepsy Behav.* 2015;53:26-30.

31. Zuberi SM, Symonds JD. Update on diagnosis and management of childhood epilepsies. *J Pediatr (Rio J).* 2015;91(6 Suppl 1):S67-S77.

32. Trost LF 3rd, Wender RC, Suter CC, et al. Management of epilepsy in adults. Treatment guidelines. *Postgrad Med.* 2005;118(6):29-33.

33. Aneja S, Sharma S. Newer anti-epileptic drugs. *Indian Pediatr.* 2013;50(11):1033-1040.

34. Johannessen Landmark C, Johannessen SI. Pharmacological management of epilepsy: recent advances and future prospects. *Drugs.* 2008;68(14):1925-1939.

35. Howard P, Twycross R, Shuster J, Mihalyo M, Remi J, Wilcock A. Anti-epileptic drugs. *J Pain Symptom Manage.* 2011;42(5):788-804.

36. Lefevre F, Aronson N. Ketogenic diet for the treatment of refractory epilepsy in children: a systematic review of efficacy. *Pediatrics.* 2000;105(4):E46.

37. Klein P, Tyrlikova I, Mathews GC. Dietary treatment in adults with refractory epilepsy: a review. *Neurology.* 2014;83(21):1978-1985.

38. Stewman CG, Liebman C, Fink L, Sandella B. Attention deficit hyperactivity disorder: unique considerations in athletes. *Sports Health.* 2018;10(1):40-46.

39. Wolfe ES, Madden KJ. Evidence-based considerations and recommendations for athletic trainers caring for patients with attention-deficit/hyperactivity disorder. *J Athl Train.* 2016;51(10):813-820.

40. Kemp S, Graham CD, Chan R, Kitchingman H, Vickerman K, Reuber M. The frequency and management of seizures during psychological treatment among patients with psychogenic nonepileptic seizures and epilepsy. *Epilepsia.* 2018;59(4):844-853.

41. Tellez-Zenteno JF, Patten SB, Jette N, Williams J, Wiebe S. Psychiatric comorbidity in epilepsy: a population-based analysis. *Epilepsia.* 2007;48(12):2336-2344.

42. Mula M, Trimble MR. Antiepileptic drug-induced cognitive adverse effects: potential mechanisms and contributing factors. *CNS Drugs.* 2009;23(2):121-137.

43. Jacoby A, Snape D, Baker GA. Determinants of quality of life in people with epilepsy. *Neurol Clin.* 2009;27(4):843-863.

44. Mohan M, Keller S, Nicolson A, et al. The long-term outcomes of epilepsy surgery. *PLoS One.* 2018;13(5):e0196274.

45. Tellez-Zenteno JF, Wiebe S. Long-term seizure and psychosocial outcomes of epilepsy surgery. *Curr Treat Options Neurol.* 2008;10(4):253-259.

46. Huizenga MN, Fureman BE, Soltesz I, Stella N. Proceedings of the Epilepsy Foundation's 2017 cannabinoids in epilepsy therapy workshop. *Epilepsy Behav.* 2018;85:237-242.

47. Stockings E, Zagic D, Campbell G, et al. Evidence for cannabis and cannabinoids for epilepsy: a systematic review of controlled and observational evidence. *J Neurol Neurosurg Psychiatry.* 2018;89(7):741-753.

48. Brodie MJ, Ben-Menachem E. Cannabinoids for epilepsy: what do we know and where do we go? *Epilepsia.* 2018;59(2):291-296.

49. Convulsive disorders and participation in sports and physical education. *JAMA.* 1968;206(6):1291.

50. Livingston S, Berman W. Participation of epileptic patients in sports. *JAMA.* 1973;224(2):236-238.

51. Pimentel J, Tojal R, Morgado J. Epilepsy and physical exercise. *Seizure.* 2015;25:87-94.

52. Corbitt RW, Cooper DL, Erickson DJ, et al. Editorial: Epileptics and contact sports. *JAMA.* 1974;229(7):820-821.

53. Sports and the child with epilepsy. *Pediatrics.* 1983;72(6):884-885.

54. ILAE Commission report. Restrictions for children with epilepsy. Commission of Pediatrics of the ILAE. International League Against Epilepsy. *Epilepsia.* 1997;38(9):1054-1056.

55. Howard GM, Radloff M, Sevier TL. Epilepsy and sports participation. *Curr Sports Med Rep.* 2004;3(1):15-19.

56. Conley KM, Bolin DJ, Carek PJ, et al. National Athletic Trainers' Association position statement: Preparticipation physical examinations and disqualifying conditions. *J Athl Train.* 2014;49(1):102-120.

57. Fountain NB, May AC. Epilepsy and athletics. *Clinics in Sports Medicine.* 2003;22(3):605-616, x-xi.

58. Miele VJ, Bailes JE, Martin NA. Participation in contact or collision sports in athletes with epilepsy, genetic risk factors, structural brain lesions, or history of craniotomy. *Neurosurg Focus.* 2006;21(4):E9.

59. Arida RM, Scorza FA, Cavalheiro EA, Perucca E, Moshe SL. Can people with epilepsy enjoy sports? *Epilepsy Res.* 2012;98(1):94-95.

60. Sahoo SK, Fountain NB. Epilepsy in football players and other land-based contact or collision sport athletes: when can they participate, and is there an increased risk? *Curr Sports Med Rep.* 2004;3(5):284-288.

61. Tellez-Zenteno JF, Hunter G, Wiebe S. Injuries in people with self-reported epilepsy: a population-based study. *Epilepsia.* 2008;49(6):954-961.

62. Vancini RL, Andrade MS, de Lira CA. Exercise as medicine for people with epilepsy. *Scand J Med Sci Sports.* 2016;26(7):856-857.

63. Volpato N, Kobashigawa J, Yasuda CL, Kishimoto ST, Fernandes PT, Cendes F. Level of physical activity and aerobic capacity associate with quality of life in patients with temporal lobe epilepsy. *PLoS One.* 2017;12(7):e0181505.

64. Allendorfer JB, Arida RM. Role of physical activity and exercise in alleviating cognitive impairment in people with epilepsy. *Clin Ther.* 2018;40(1):26-34.

65. Wirth M, Haase CM, Villeneuve S, Vogel J, Jagust WJ. Neuroprotective pathways: lifestyle activity, brain pathology, and cognition in cognitively normal older adults. *Neurobiol Aging.* 2014;35(8):1873-1882.

66. Parks ED. Seizure disorders in athletes. *Athl Ther Today.* 2006;11(4):36-38.

67. Epilepsy Foundation. Seizure First Aid and Safety. https://www.epilepsy.com/learn/seizure-first-aid-and-safety/tailoring-first-aid-plans. Accessed September 11, 2018.

68. Seizure Response Plans 101. Epilepsy Foundation. https://www.epilepsy.com/learn/managing-your-epilepsy/seizure-response-plans-101. Accessed September 11, 2018.

69. Aneja S. Benzodiazepines for acute management of seizures. *Indian J Pediatr.* 2012;79(3):381-382.

70. Cherian A, Thomas SV. Status epilepticus. *Ann Indian Acad Neurol.* 2009;12(3):140-153.

71. Maglalang PD, Rautiola D, Siegel RA, et al. Rescue therapies for seizure emergencies: new modes of administration. *Epilepsia.* 2018;59 Suppl2:207-215.

72. Hartman AL, Devore CD. Rescue medicine for epilepsy in education settings. *Pediatrics.* 2016;137(1).

73. Collard SS, Ellis-Hill C. 'I'd rather you didn't come': the impact of stigma on exercising with epilepsy. *J Health Psychol.* 2017:1359105317729560.

11

Psychiatric Issues

Christian Conte, PhD and Donald J. Conte, MS, MA

CHAPTER KEY WORDS

- Conscious education
- Exploring options
- Suicidal ideation
- Yield theory

CHAPTER SCENARIO

Brian, a running back on the football team, moved halfway across the country to be at your university. A standout athlete since he first started playing the game, Brian was an all-conference player as a freshman, then got a season-ending knee injury at the start of his sophomore year. He worked hard in rehab, but when he got back out onto the field in the first game of his junior season, he endured a season-ending shoulder injury. By his senior year, another running back was an all-star for the team, which dropped Brian on the depth chart. This had a tremendous impact on Brian because he went from being an all-conference player as a freshman to being a backup as a senior, all due to injuries. Two weeks into this season, Brian sustained a concussion, which put him out of play for the following week.

His coaches, teammates, your colleagues, and you all noticed drastic changes in Brian's demeanor. For example, as a freshman, he was probably best described as the life of the party, but now he was significantly quieter, and he seemed to be angry more frequently. You notice that he has become more agitated and irritable recently, and he

disclosed that he and his girlfriend of 2 years recently split. When you make a comment validating Brian's tough situation, he responds by saying, "I don't care. I don't even want to be here anymore," and then shuts down, not wanting to offer anything else.

SCENARIO RESOLUTION

Now that you know him and both his athletic and personal history to some extent, you are, whether or not you want to be, a part of his situation. Your challenge is to identify whether or not Brian has a psychiatric emergency and would benefit from a referral to a mental health service.

INTRODUCTION

The idea of being responsible for someone else's emotional and psychological well-being can sound intimidating and overwhelming, especially for those with limited training in the field of psychology and counseling. However, the good news is that, as an athletic trainer, you are not responsible for anyone else's emotional and psychological well-being. In fact, even if you were a psychologist or counselor, that statement would still be true.

However, you are responsible for the part you play in every communication you have, and, as a professional, you are responsible for identifying when to refer an athlete to counseling or mental health support services. In short, as

Feld F., Gorse KM, Blanc RO
Non-Orthopedic Emergency Care in Athletics (pp 89-97).
© 2020 Taylor & Francis Group.

in any profession in which you work with others, you are always responsible for identifying whether something constitutes a psychiatric emergency.

Injuries can leave anyone feeling vulnerable, and athletes are no exception. From a state of vulnerability, athletes often share personal issues with their trainers. When athletes open up, you have 2 primary areas of focus: identifying psychological issues that require referral and navigating your part of the communication with them. In this chapter, we'll show you how to both identify psychological challenges in others and communicate effectively with people, regardless of any issue they might be facing.

The first message to learn regarding handling athletes' psychological issues is this: You do not have to fix anyone. You only have to effectively listen to them to clearly identify what they are communicating. Identifying issues as problematic becomes easier when you set aside the need, desire, or pressure to solve what others are experiencing and instead focus on being accurate in your understanding of what they're conveying. Perhaps the simplest guideline for recognizing whether an issue is worthy of referral is this: any issue that interferes with a person's daily functioning is problematic.

Psychological distress is not a sign of weakness. All humans experience psychological struggles from time to time, and injuries that disrupt the projected or expected course of athletes' lives can certainly weigh on them psychologically. The culture of sports has traditionally discouraged signs of weakness, and while equating psychological distress with weakness is unfortunate and inaccurate, the history of sport culture, coupled with popular understanding of mental health, perpetuates the association. Although many of us in the mental health field have been fighting against this stigma and false association for a long time, it can be the cultural context and the perceived reality of any athlete under stress. The more you align your expectations about your role with the reality of this unfortunate stigma, the more prepared you will be to accurately meet athletes where they are psychologically and to help guide them through any barriers that might impede them from seeking mental health support.

One possible approach to normalize the process of athletes following through with counseling services lies in comparing the roles of sports psychologists, who demonstrably help athletes and teams improve their performance, with the roles of mental health practitioners, who can be thought of as psychological or mental coaches who help people navigate difficult emotional situations.

Any time you put the pressure of solving others' problems on your shoulders, you place an unnecessary and unrealistic burden on yourself. In contrast, when you recognize that your responsibility is simply to approach others with compassion, with a nonjudgmental attitude, authentic humility, and genuine curiosity to learn about them, you allay the pressure to solve their problems. In addition, you create a psychologically safe environment that enables others to express themselves openly and honestly and share their inner, subjective experience. The more honest others are about what they're experiencing in the unseen world of their minds, the more accurately you can assess their need for help. By approaching others in this way, you also open a path for them to help themselves by working through their emotions, following through with mental health referrals, or initiating whatever other approach may be helpful.

This chapter first looks at the nature of Yield Theory, a pragmatic approach for helping you communicate with athletes and identify potential psychiatric emergencies, and then demonstrates its use in a case such as Brian's.

Yield Theory

The hands-on, pragmatic method that we present in this chapter for helping you communicate with athletes in the most intentional way possible is called *Yield Theory*. Yield Theory is a powerful form of connecting with others, rooted in compassion and conscious education. It is an evidenced-based approach that will help you circumvent others' fight-or-flight responses (ie, their defensiveness and resistance) to help them identify the heart of their challenges in a straightforward, yet nonthreatening way.[1] In other words, Yield Theory helps you communicate with others in a way that makes them feel safe enough to let their guard down and tell you what is really going on. By providing you with a simple yet effective methodology for communication, we hope you will learn how to approach every professional discussion with intentionality.

Yield Theory takes the concept of walking a mile in others' shoes a step further and invites you to take a moment to visualize yourself *as* the other person talking to you, complete with that person's cognitive functioning, ability to experience emotions, and life experiences. When you put yourself behind others' eyes, it wipes away the tendency for you to listen through the filter of what you believe you would do if you were them. You can set aside biases, preconceived notions, and judgment to focus on assessing what is going on. To accomplish seeing the world as others see it, Yield Theory involves genuinely meeting people at their juncture by using 3 core actions that are ultimately rooted in 7 fundamental components. The 3 core actions are:

1. Listen
2. Validate
3. Explore options

The 7 fundamental components are:

1. Acceptance
2. Authenticity
3. Compassion
4. Conscious education
5. Creativity

6. Mindfulness

7. Nonattachment

The idea of listening, validating, and exploring options is simple to understand and pragmatic to use—but that is not necessarily easy-to-do. As an analogy, think of the greatest martial artists in the history of the world. Ultimately, their 3 core actions are move, block, and hit, but, as you know, there is great skill in the way they move, block, and hit. Similarly, all great communicators listen, validate, and explore options, but it is how they listen, validate, and explore options that makes all the difference.

Just as it takes practice to become a master martial artist, it takes practice to become a great communicator. By focusing on the technique of how to listen, validate, and explore options with proficiency, you will learn how to connect with others in a deep and meaningful way, even if only during a brief interaction. Through being intentional with your approach, you will learn how to quickly assess whether you need to refer an athlete to mental health professionals for additional support.

Listen

Becoming an effective listener takes practice, but there are ways to increase your ability. To listen to others is to hear the entirety of what they are communicating. Barriers, such as ego or pride, often get in the way of listening well. The ego expects others to match its perspective, making us focus on what we believe others *should* or *will* say, rather on what they *do* say. For instance, it is natural for one to assume, but making assumptions about what others are communicating can lead to inaccurate assessments and miscommunication. Moreover, holding fast to assumptions stems from our ego's desire to know, be right, or be seen as the expert. The challenge effective listeners face is to set aside their ego and listen for what is actually being communicated. It takes a certain level of self-awareness as well as the humility for having the willingness to learn about the person.

A useful analogy for listening effectively is to imagine that you are standing on one side of an enormous building, and the people with whom you are communicating are standing on the other side. There is no way for you to understand what is going on over there, because you cannot see what is happening, so you have to listen intently to what those people describe they are seeing and experiencing. Instead of listening to correct them and tell them what you believe they are seeing, you would listen openly with the singular desire of learning what they see and experience.

In considering this analogy, you allow yourself to recognize that you simply cannot see what you are not able to see—the interior, subjective world of the speaker. To listen in this way is to do so without judgment, with the humility and genuine sense of curiosity that drives your desire to learn. Think of communication with someone as a learning experience in which the other person is the teacher and you are the eager student.

Just as you cannot simultaneously see 2 opposite sides of a large building while standing on one side, seeing into the inner subjective world of others is equally as impossible. In both instances, listening involves accepting others' perceptions of their experience. People are not wrong or bad for their feelings, and we cannot tell them what they experience in their own minds. However, what we can do is listen openly. From the position of, "Teach me about what you're experiencing," we are in a much better place to show others the kind of interest that is likely to lead to their opening up and being honest about what they're experiencing. The more open and honest others are about what is going on inside them, the more accurately you can assess the situation.

Listening to Content Versus Process

When it comes to communication, there is a difference between content and process. Content comprises the words people say, whereas process comprises the manner of speech. When a there is a discrepancy between people's emotions and behavior, it is an indicator that something more is going on psychologically than what they are ready to disclose or what they are aware or unaware of personally. For instance, the response, "I'm fine" can have multiple meanings, depending on the tone the speaker uses, as shown in the following examples:

- "I'm fine," he said, annoyed.
- "I'm fine," he said angrily.
- "I'm fine," he said reassuringly.
- "I'm fine," he said indifferently.

In each case, when the person says, "I'm fine," the meaning is different. In all the cases except one, the process is different from the content. When you listen to others, it is important to listen to both content and process. The bigger the discrepancy, the more likely that something more is going on internally.

There are two creative ways to quickly identify process: (1) imagine that you are seeing that person speak, but the sound is on mute, so you are solely watching the person's body language and facial expressions and/or (2) to imagine that the person could use only one word to share what she or he wanted to express, and that one word likely comprises the person's process.

When people speak, they are communicating, both with what they tell you and what their body language, tone, and facial expressions show you. To listen to athletes well is to distinguish between their content and process, and then to recognize which of the 2 is more emphatic. An athlete can tell you that she is okay, but her body language and actions can show you that she is more upset than she is willing to reveal. One reason people do not readily reveal what is going on deep in their emotional worlds is that they, like you, want to feel psychologically safe before they allow themselves to be vulnerable enough to open up.

One of the best ways to help others feel safe enough to open up is by conveying interest and nonjudgment. The pragmatic tool of compassion for communicating interest without judgment is validation.

Validate

Once you have listened to what others say and believe you have identified their process, the second step in the process of Yield Theory is to validate. To validate is to acknowledge how others feel. To validate others' emotions is not to condone their actions; it is simply to fully acknowledge the emotions they report they have. The more authentic you are in expressing interest in others and validating with compassion, the safer others feel, and the more likely they are to be honest about what they're experiencing in their inner, subjective worlds.

Making a statement of validation in many ways can be thought of as a self-check. Through validation, you are checking to see whether you have accurately heard what others are expressing. Saying something like, "You seem angry" allows the other person to either confirm your hypothesis or correct you. In general, statements of validation might begin with "You seem . . ." or "It sounds like you feel . . ." or just a statement that you are identifying the emotion the other person is expressing. The more you listen with humility, the less attached you'll be to your response derived from your own thoughts and feelings.

Validation is a focus on the perspective others are sharing that can circumvent their defensiveness. The more others feel understood, the more they feel connected. The more connected we feel with others, the safer we feel—remember, safety is the key to circumventing the fight, flight, or freeze response.

Once people feel validated, they are ready to explore options, but a common mistake communicators often make is rushing a person to explore options when he or she might still be in an emotional state that requires listening and validating. Although the brain is a complex of interacting neurons, problem-solving and emoting largely occur in 2 unique areas of the brain. To help people get to the part of the problem-solving center of their brain that will help them make clear decisions, you want to listen and validate them until they feel validated, not just until you feel you have validated them. Although you can begin to explore options while people are in a heightened emotional state, the general rule of thumb is to validate others until you can see a shift in their nonverbal communication, which indicates they have at least released some energy via your validation.

Explore Options

When people are struggling emotionally and say extreme things, there is a tendency for listeners to get swept up in the content of what others say and react to it. For example, if an athlete says out of frustration, "I should just quit!" then those around her might respond, "No, you don't want to do that." A quick, stereotypical response like that is reflective of minimizing and downplaying that athlete's emotional experience. It also indicates a failure to realize that what people say in intense emotional states might not be what they actually want to do. Getting swept up in the content of what people say can be misleading, just as you have not always meant what you said in high emotional states. However, instead of focusing in on the content of what others disclose, it is more important for you to focus on the process of what they're communicating.

The way to do that is to not resist any potential choice they express. The options people mention in intense emotional states are often more indicative of their process or emotional state than of their actual desire. Of course, that is not a hard rule, as sometimes people want to do exactly what they say they will do in extreme emotional states. Again, the goal is to ascertain what others are genuinely communicating and to discern what is being emphasized more—content or process.

No matter what an athlete shares with you regarding potential options, yielding entails going with or verbally playing out that option with compassion, rather than resisting or denying it as a choice. In other words, if someone thinks it, then it is an option for him or her. That does not mean you have to agree with all potential options or that you cannot express an opinion about which option you believe is best. What it does mean is that by not resisting the options people give you, you will have a better chance to meet others where they are, not where you or others might believe they should be.

For example, telling the athlete who says she should quit that quitting is not an option would be the opposite of Yield Theory. Quitting is, in fact, an option, and may be the only one she entertains at the moment. However, you can acknowledge that her personal choice does not have to be the end of the conversation; rather, it is only a starting point for exploring the options she has not yet considered. The more emotional people are regarding a topic, the fewer options they tend to see for themselves, which is why, as a neutral observer, you can show the troubled athlete that more options do exist.

The more time you have to explore options with someone, the more you can play out their ideas to conclusion. So, regarding quitting, you could say, "Okay, so let's say you quit. That's definitely an option, and if I'm in your shoes, I can see why I might also want to explore that. So, let's say you do quit, then what do you plan to do?" Without judging the options that others are considering, you take away the need for them to defend that path of action. Through nonresistance, you can create a safe space psychologically for people to share whatever they need to share.

Again, your goal is not to analyze, diagnose, or treat the psychiatric struggle that you recognize, but it is important for you to recognize what is happening as you communicate clearly and compassionately with the athletes you treat physically. Without downplaying or ignoring what the athlete expresses, keep in mind that whatever option others share with you, it is real and viable in their eyes. By acknowledging their stated options and the feelings and attitudes associated with them, you circumvent their innate desire to defend those options. Whatever option people express, assume that it is realistic, and be prepared to earnestly play out what following through with that option might look like.

For another example, let's say that an athlete expresses his anger to you about another player "disrespecting him" in the locker room earlier that day. The enraged athlete says that he is considering fighting his teammate. Instead of telling him that it is unwise from a Yield Theory perspective of nonresistance, it is more important to imagine that you were in his place and that you were having an identical emotional response. In that way, you can listen openly to what he has to say without resistance and validate how he feels. Nonresistance does not refer to your condoning anything others say they're going to do, rather, it means that you do not resist or tell others how they feel or what they should or should not be saying or single out the only option you feel is effective. By listening to this athlete's experience and validating his anger, you make yourself a safe psychological space in which he is significantly more likely to both be honest about what he is genuinely considering doing and more willing to listen to you play out what it would look like if he actually followed through with that option.

You: "Okay, so let's say you fight him, then what happens?"

Athlete: "Then he learns his lesson not to mess with me."

You: "It's hard to feel like people are messing with you."

Athlete: "I'm sick of him messing with me."

You: "I can't imagine."

Once the athlete feels you care and are not resisting what he is considering, he is significantly more likely to accept your exploring other potential options with him.

You: "So, let's say that you fight him. You win. You beat him. Now what?"

Athlete: "Now the coach kicks me off the team."

You: "Okay, and maybe that's not worth it to you. Maybe it is."

Athlete: "I don't care!"

You: "I get that. And maybe you don't. Now. But I'm just wondering what the 'you' who's around 6 months from now will think. And I'm wondering what the 'you' a year from now will think. It just seems to me that if

you choose to fight him, you are basically giving him the control of your future, and if he already bothers you now, I can't imagine how much it will bother you if he determines your future in this sport."

By not resisting the athlete's anger, you can legitimately explore viable options with him. Understanding what constitutes a viable option is very important. Just because a decision is ineffective, irresponsible, or not preferable, it does not make it unviable. The basis of Yield Theory is this: if people are already considering a decision, then pretending it is not real or possible is not realistic. It is more effective from a Yield Theory perspective to acknowledge the decisions that people are considering than to deny that the decisions are feasible simply because they are uncomfortable for you or unreasonable in your eyes. Remember: your goal is to see the world through the other person's eyes.

Options do not have to be complex. Sometimes the options an athlete faces are whether to tell a parent that they reinjured themselves in a minor injury. However, other times the options athletes face center on potentially life-altering problems. Consider the athlete who is weighing the option of telling someone about a teammate who is consistently breaking team rules, or, much more seriously, the athlete who is considering whether or not he should follow through with his suicidal ideations. By moving through this 3-step process of listening, validating, and exploring options, you have the potential to identify whether others are experiencing a psychiatric emergency and/or could benefit from a mental health referral.

The Seven Fundamental Components

Yield Theory's 7 fundamental components provide a way to listen, validate, and explore options while circumventing others' defensiveness. Being able to articulate the greatest advice in the world is meaningless if the person with whom you're speaking does not hear what you have to say. These 7 fundamental components also serve as a way to provide a safe environment that allows you to communicate effectively—that is, in a way that is actually heard. These components can best be thought of as spokes on a wheel—they all converge on the central hub. The following brief overview of the 7 components provides a backdrop for how you can listen, validate, and explore options in the most effective way possible.

The first component, **acceptance**, refers to meeting others where they are. Specifically, it connotes accepting without trying to minimize or downplay what others are saying. Often, when communication is centered on uncomfortable topics, people tend to gloss over or ignore whatever they find unpleasant. Unfortunately, this tendency inhibits people from acknowledging the reality perceived by someone who is enclosed by depression or beset by suicidal thoughts. To accept where others are is not equivalent to condoning what they might say or tolerating any intolerable harmful actions. Instead, acceptance requires you to understand that, just like you, others believe their feelings are significant and, in some instances, possibly life-altering. Acceptance also refers to recognizing and accepting others' readiness and willingness to change. People "are where they are" in attitude, emotion, and knowledge and the sooner we recognize where others are, the more efficiently we will be able to meet them there.

The second component, **authenticity**, requires you to be genuine in your interactions. Because people can easily identify when others are genuinely interested in them, it is important to be authentic regarding the way you express care and concern for others. Thus, a key to authenticity is self-awareness. For example, through self-awareness, you can be aware of whether or not there is a congruence between your own content and process. Authenticity occurs when your content and process match, so if you express care and concern, others will be able to see that care and concern in your nonverbal behaviors as well. Authenticity is a pathway to clear and harmonious communication.

The third component is **compassion**. Compassion literally means *to suffer with*, and leading with compassion is the primary way you can circumvent others' defensiveness. Although we can only ever experience life through our individual experience, feeling connected to others alleviates suffering, even if in some minor way. The more you lead with compassion, the less judgmental you are and the more you can assume an authentic nonjudgmental demeanor that connects you to others. A compassionate connection engenders a feeling of safety that opens others to be honest about their thoughts and feelings. By leading with compassion, you will be in a better position to make a more accurate assessment of others' otherwise hidden, subjective realities, and get to the heart of any potential psychiatric emergency.

The fourth component is **conscious education**. Conscious education centers on expanding others' awareness. Anytime people are experiencing intense emotions, their ability to explore options becomes significantly narrowed. The more information you can contribute to others, the more you can expand their awareness. Conscious education technically occurs anytime you add information to others' lives. It can be as simple as helping others see that every emotional situation, no matter how intense, will have a beginning, middle, and end, and that it is wise not to make an impulsive decision in the beginning or middle of a situation that results in an unwanted long-term consequence. In that case, conscious education involves helping athletes see that essentially, "this too shall pass." Bringing that kind of awareness to the present moment might seem to be a simplistic approach, but it has profound consequences because it gives the athlete a chance to step back to assess his or her options without the irritability, anger, and feeling of hopelessness that often accompany an injury.

The fifth component is **creativity**. Creativity is fundamental because people learn in different ways, and if the goal in clear communication is to meet others where they are and help them expand awareness, then doing so

creatively gives you a better chance to meet diverse learners where they are. Sometimes creativity means using anecdotes, analogies and metaphors to enhance communication and to make a point that resonates with the athlete. An athlete whose negative emotions center on being "disrespected" by fans, coaches, or teammates, might benefit from a marionette analogy: Allowing another to control how one feels (e.g., angry, sad, humiliated), makes one into a puppet whose strings another pulls. The analogy can elicit in the athlete a desire to break free from the control of another person or group. Because there is no limit to creativity, Yield Theory encourages every athletic trainer to treat each athlete as an individual, and that means using creative approaches. Such anecdotes, analogies, and metaphors should be brief and easy to understand. For example, drawing on popular culture, a trainer could point out that Iron Man's power is buried in his chest and that the superhero would not take his power source out and hand it over to another, especially to one who wanted to control him. Handing over one's "super power" (i.e., relinquishing control over emotions) is what anyone does in acquiescing to peer pressure and "disrespect."

The sixth component is **mindfulness**, which can simply be understood as awareness. Mindfulness in terms of communication is profoundly important. First, it is crucial for you to be mindful of your presence. From the distance you are to others, to the tone of your voice, facial expressions, and body language, people see your actions, not your intentions. The more mindful you are of how you come across to others, as well as what others bring out of you, the better you can adjust what you need to when the moment comes. Second, it is critical to be mindful of the difference between others' content and process, as well as whether or not others are in immediate danger. Mindfulness is an ongoing process that is best enhanced through a focus on presence. The more in tune with the present you can be, the more mindful you will be.

The seventh component is **nonattachment**. Nonattachment refers to the separation between you and your thoughts and emotions. For example, the more attached you are to what you say, the more likely you are to get upset when others disagree with you. Nonattachment is especially important in listening, validating, and exploring options. In terms of listening, the less attached you are to your preconceived notions, the more open you'll be to listening to what others are actually communicating, instead of hearing only what you believed you would hear. In terms of validation, the less attached you are to your statements of validation, the more quickly you can readjust to reflect the corrections others make. In regard to exploring options, nonattachment is perhaps most important because the less attached you are to the options that you suggest, the less others are likely to resist having to follow through with what you say and the more likely they are to genuinely explore the options you present.

Identifying and Handling Suicidal Ideations

Death is a scary subject for many, and suicide is perhaps even more so because it appears to take the lives of seemingly healthy and well-adjusted people. Suicide most often occurs when stressors and health issues converge to create an experience of hopelessness and despair. However, suicide is preventable, and there are often warning signs. There are also risk factors.

Some of the warning signs of suicide include talking about dying; expressing hopelessness and feelings of entrapment; experiencing "unbearable" pain; using drugs and/or alcohol in increasing amounts; withdrawing from activities and previous positive behaviors; searching for ways to end life; and showing signs of depression, anxiety, loss of interest, humiliation, and shame. Each of us is complex, so these motivations for suicide can be combined or other motivations can be involved.

People who are at the highest level of risk for suicide generally tend to have a plan, have access to complete that plan, then do not have reasons to stop them from following through with their plan. For instance, if a person has thought through that he or she would use a gun, has access to a gun, and has no reason to stop from following through, then he or she would be at the highest risk. If, on the other hand, a person expresses a vague sense of not wanting to be alive anymore but has no plan and also has strong religious beliefs against committing suicide, then he or she is at a lower risk (although the person still should be taken seriously). Any athlete who expresses suicidal ideations should be referred to mental health services.

It is important to approach people who express suicidal ideations with compassion and nonjudgment. It is also imperative that you get additional support for someone with a suicidal mindset. The nature of suicidal ideations is such that you cannot let apprehensions interfere with your getting immediate support for the suicidal person. In many instances, the awkwardness in a discussion about suicide occurs in the listener, not in the person contemplating suicide. The latter might feel relief that he or she can talk to a compassionate listener in a safe, nonjudgmental environment. For those who think about suicide, judgment and shame do not provide any relief or reconsideration. They need to express what they are experiencing internally. That means that you need to do whatever it takes to work through your own discomfort or uneasiness; your connection to someone with suicidal ideation can literally be lifesaving.

Both the Centers for Disease Control and Prevention and the US Food and Drug Administration have published studies on suicidal ideation.[3] The common ground between these agencies regarding suicidal ideation is a set of 5 conditions, or risk factors, the last of which puts a person at highest risk. These conditions are:

1. Passive (no active intent, plan, or method associated with suicidal ideation)
2. Active: Nonspecific (no intent, plan, or method)
3. Active: Method but no intent or plan
4. Active: Method and intent but no plan
5. Active: Method, intent, and plan[2]

With respect to an athlete with suicidal ideation, your job as an athletic trainer is essentially to recognize the need for professional mental health aid. Regardless of which condition might apply to an athlete, you should recognize that suicidal ideation is a possibly strong motivator that could result in self-harm.

Applying Yield Theory to Brian

When it comes to applying Yield Theory to the case of Brian, the first thing to remember is the 3 core actions: listen, validate, and explore options. To listen to Brian is to really get into his phenomenological world and try to understand what it would be like to be him. Imagine yourself having experienced the number and depths of injuries he experienced, including the shift his identity would have taken after going from an all-star to a backup. On top of these on-field struggles, imagine also that you lost a relationship that was meaningful to you. Finally, picture yourself being far from your core family.

The important piece in listening to keep in your foreground is this—you are not just picturing your own life. For instance, even if you are away from your family, you will not have the exact same family relationships, and it will not mean the same thing to you that it means to Brian. Instead, you are trying to visualize Brian's life as Brian sees it.

Imagine that you do listen and validate Brian, and he gets to the point at the end of the scenario when he says, "I don't care. I don't even want to be here anymore." The most pressing information to find out is what he means by "here." Does "here" mean on the football team, or at the university, or living? To effectively assess whether or not Brian is in the middle of a psychiatric emergency or in need of a mental health referral, it is important to continue with listening, validating, and exploring options.

First, listen to Brian describe his situation without making any assumptions. Be mindful that there is no one right way to have experiences and that he is justified in feeling anything he feels. Listen to Brian as though he is standing on the other side of a big building, and the only way for you to understand what he is seeing on that side of the building is to listen with humility, completely setting your ego aside.

Next, validate Brian's feelings. Again, it is important to understand that validating how Brian feels is not condoning what might be anything from potentially quitting the football team, to leaving school, or worse, legitimate suicidal ideations. Validate Brian until he feels validated. You will be able to tell that he feels validated by watching his nonverbal communication, but you can be most assured he feels validated by his verbally acknowledging that he feels understood. Sometimes people say things along the lines of, "I feel like you really understand where I'm coming from," or "I appreciate your listening because you seem to get what I'm saying." These are just some of the many statements that can indicate a person feels validated. When Brian begins to feel validated, you can start to explore options with him.

Finally, as you explore options with Brian, make sure you are continually listening to him and validating him. You obviously do not have to repeat to him or reflect everything he says. Truly effective communication is an art form, and no rote series of statements can fit for all people and all situations. The general guideline is to be humble regarding the way you listen, be compassionate regarding the way you validate, and be realistic regarding the way you explore options. The options that Brian discusses are *options*, even if they seem unpleasant, so start by exploring those. The more accepting you are of Brian's ideas, the more likely he is to be honest about what he is actually thinking.

At a minimum, based on everything Brian has experienced over the past couple years, it would be beneficial for him to talk to a counselor. Again, phrasing this as having a "mental coach" or just someone in a neutral position to provide insight is a helpful way to normalize the process of counseling. The more you genuinely see human behavior on a continuum, the more you will truly believe yourself that counseling is a process of insight from which anyone can benefit because mental health counselors are trained to listen, validate, and explore options in diverse ways and with sound methodology.[4]

Be assured that not every approach works with everyone and that no approach you take indicates a failure on your part to change someone. Ultimately, everyone has responsibility for his or her own thoughts and behaviors. Your primary concern is the well-being of those in your care to the extent that you are authentic as you listen, validate, and explore options. The more you can practice the basics of Yield Theory, the more prepared you'll be to handle any potential psychiatric emergency that might come your way.

CHAPTER SUMMARY

Often, athletes open up to their trainers in the normal course of conversation during treatment. When people are injured or vulnerable physically, they often also feel vulnerable mentally. Although it is not in your scope of practice as an athletic trainer to treat mental health complications, it is well within your profession to identify and refer athletes when applicable. When issues begin to interfere with normal functioning, those issues become problematic. The intentional approach to communication presented in this chapter is Yield Theory, which is a method of communication rooted in compassion and conscious education and centered in the 3 core actions of listening, validating, and exploring options.

CHAPTER REVIEW QUESTIONS

1. Explain the difference between validating and condoning.
2. What part of the brain acts as a center for emotions?
3. What is difference between ego-centered and other-centered listening?
4. Why would the following response to a troubled athlete be ineffective? "I know how you feel. When I played, I ran into a similar problem."
5. What is the goal of validation?

ANSWERS

1. Validating is a form of empathizing. It is a nonjudgmental acknowledgment that someone else's feelings or perspective are real for that person and a motive for his or her behavior. Condoning is a form of complicit justification of another's behavior. It is also a form of agreeing with another person's ideas or behaviors.
2. (Short answer) The limbic system. (Long answer) The brain is a complex of many connected systems, but the limbic system in the brain's interior is the seat of emotions.
3. In ego-centered listening, one sees from his or her perspective and life experiences, not from the perspective and experiences of another. Ego-centered listeners make declarative statements. An ego-centered listener might say something like, "Yes, I understand. I had a similar experience . . ." Other-centered listening places the emphasis on what the other person expresses from his or her perspective and experiences. Other-centered listeners say something similar to the question "Could you tell me more about that?" Other-centered listeners ask perceptive questions to learn more about the other person.
4. The response would be an ego-centered one that puts the emphasis not on the athlete and his or her problem, but rather on the listener's experiences.
5. The goal of validation is to drain the limbic system to allow a more cerebral approach to a problem.

REFERENCES

1. Conte C. *Advanced Techniques for Counseling and Psychotherapy.* New York, NY: Springer Publishing Company; 2009.

2. US Food and Drug Administration. Center for Drug Evaluation and Research. Guidances (Drugs) - Guidance for Industry: Suicidal Ideation and Behavior: Prospective Assessment of Occurrence in Clinical Trials. https://www.fda.gov/Drugs/GuidanceComplianceRegulatoryInformation/Guidances/ucm315156.htm. Accessed June 20, 2019.

3. Crosby AE, Ortega L, and Melanson C. *Self-Directed Violence Surveillance: Uniform Definitions and Recommended Data Elements.* Centers for Disease Control and Prevention, National Center for Injury Prevention and Control, Division of Violence Prevention. Published 2011. https://www.cdc.gov/violenceprevention/pdf/Self-Directed-Violence-a.pdf. Accessed October 3, 2018.

4. Conte C. *Walking through Anger: A New Design for Confronting Conflict in an Emotionally Charged World.* Boulder, CO: Sounds True, Inc; 2019

12

Abdominal Emergencies

Harsh K. Desai, MD; Christine M. Leeper, MD; and Kevin Garrett, MD

CHAPTER KEY WORDS

- Blunt abdominal trauma
- Hollow viscus injury
- Solid-organ injury

CHAPTER SCENARIO

An 18-year-old male was elbowed in his left upper quadrant while playing soccer at a tournament several hours from his home. He continued to play and returned home at the conclusion of the game, but presented to the hospital 5 hours later with increasing abdominal pain, nausea, and weakness. His vital signs included blood pressure 98/54, pulse 80, oxygen saturation 100%, and respiratory rate 20. On examination, he was pale, diaphoretic, and had moderate tenderness to palpation in the left upper quadrant. A bedside ultrasound showed free fluid in the abdomen (Figure 12-1). Two large-bore intravenous catheters were placed, and 2 L of crystalloid fluid was administered with improvement in blood pressure. He underwent a computed tomography scan of his abdomen and pelvis with contrast, which revealed a splenic laceration in the lower pole of the spleen, active contrast extravasation from a branch of the splenic artery, and moderate hemoperitoneum (Figure 12-2).

SCENARIO RESOLUTION

The patient was transferred to a trauma center, where he underwent exploratory laparotomy and splenectomy (Figure 12-3). No other injuries were identified, and the patient was admitted to a monitored surgical floor. He recovered uneventfully and was discharged to home on post-trauma day 4, at which time he was eating a regular diet, ambulating, and performing all activities independently. He was instructed to resume daily activities gradually and return to cardio training in 3 to 4 weeks. He was cleared for weight lifting and sports contact after 8 weeks.

INTRODUCTION

Abdominal pain in athletes has a broad differential diagnosis. Pain may be an indication of life-threatening injury (eg, a splenic laceration), acute illness (eg, appendicitis), or more benign causes (eg, soft tissue bruising or muscle cramping). Evaluation of the athlete with abdominal pain should include a focused history regarding pain characteristics (eg, onset, duration, migration, and alleviating or exacerbating factors), antecedent trauma, and associated symptoms (eg, fever, vomiting, and weakness). Examination of the abdomen includes inspection for signs of trauma (eg, ecchymosis, abrasions, and lacerations) as well as superficial and deep palpation to assess for tenderness or peritonitis. If there is concern for significant injury, 911 should be activated to expedite evaluation in the

Feld F., Gorse KM, Blanc RO
Non-Orthopedic Emergency Care in Athletes (pp 99-104)
© 2020 Taylor & Francis Group.

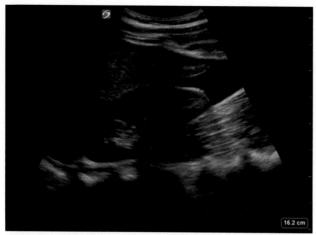

Figure 12-1. Bedside ultrasound demonstrates free fluid within the abdomen adjacent to the kidney and liver.

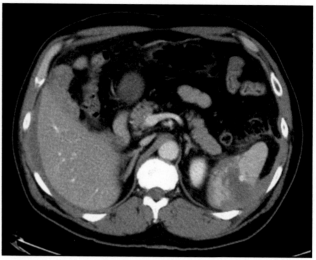

Figure 12-2. CT scan of the abdomen demonstrates splenic injury.

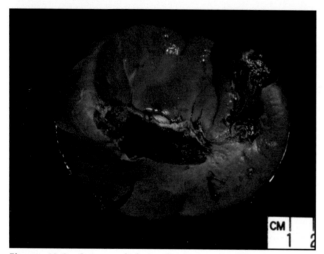

Figure 12-3. Gross pathology demonstrates splenic laceration post-splenectomy.

appropriate setting. Athletes should refrain from eating or drinking prior to medical evaluation, and medical professionals should withhold pain medications to allow for a reliable physical examination.

Survival is improved when injured patients receive care at a designated trauma center—whether adult, pediatric, or combined—as compared to a non-trauma center. Further, pediatric patients have increased survival when cared for at designated pediatric trauma centers.[1-3] Although most patients without serious injury can be evaluated and cared for in their local medical centers, they may be stabilized and transferred to a specialized center if they have significant injury mechanism, significant injury burden (eg, multiple long-bone fractures, polytrauma, amputation, spinal cord injury, spine fracture, severe head, polytrauma), or if they require specialist services at a tertiary care center.[4]

Solid-Organ Injury

Evaluation

Solid-organ injury is common in athletes after significant blunt abdominal trauma. The spleen is the most commonly injured solid organ (25% to 39%), followed by the liver (15% to 37%), kidney (19% to 25%), and pancreas (7%).[5] While splenic injury is more common than hepatic injury, damage to the liver is responsible for most fatal solid-organ injuries and can result in significant hemorrhage and massive blood loss. Solid-organ injury should be suspected based on physical examination findings and injury mechanism. Injury mechanism, such as abrupt deceleration, impact from the handlebar of a bicycle or all-terrain vehicle, or trauma from a direct blow to the abdomen, should raise suspicion for intra-abdominal injury.

Determining which patients need a CT scan is an area of active research interest, particularly in adolescents and young adults. The desire to limit radiation burden should be weighed against the risk of missing significant intra-abdominal injury. Patients with evidence of abdominal wall or torso trauma on physical examination, with complaints of abdominal pain or presence of abdominal tenderness, vomiting, abnormal laboratory studies (eg, alanine aminotransferase and aspartate aminotransferase >200/125, elevated amylase/lipase, 100 renal plasma clearance on urinalysis), gross hematuria, or a positive bedside ultrasound should undergo additional imaging with contrasted CT scan if hemodynamically stable versus fluid resuscitation and/or operative intervention if hemodynamically unstable. Patients without these signs and symptoms are at low risk for intra-abdominal injury and can likely be observed without additional imaging or intervention.[6]

Management

Immediate operative intervention is indicated in patients with peritonitis or hemodynamic instability. If a trial of nonoperative management is attempted, failure of this strategy is signified by worsening abdominal examination, ongoing blood transfusion requirements, or hemodynamic instability.[7] Surgical intervention for splenic injury typically involves a total splenectomy, although other alternatives include partial splenectomy or splenorrhaphy. Hepatic injury can sometimes be controlled with cautery, application of hemostasis agents, and drainage. Nonanatomic resections or formal lobectomies are required less often. Kidney injury requires operative intervention for patients with hemodynamic instability, expanding retroperitoneal hematoma, vascular pedicle injury, urinomas, or major renal vascular injury.[4] Pancreatic injury is uncommon, and optimal management is debated among experts (Figure 12-3). For blunt pancreatic injuries, major factors guiding management decisions include the presence of ductal injury and its location (ie, proximal vs distal). In the setting of duct injury, options include partial pancreatectomy for distal duct injuries and conservative interventions (eg, closed suction drainage and endoscopic stenting) for proximal ductal injuries.[8]

In patients who are unstable, surgical management often includes a damage control strategy. Surgical bleeding and gross fecal contamination are addressed expeditiously, packs are placed to tamponade coagulopathic bleeding, temporary closure of the abdomen is performed, and patients are stabilized and resuscitated in the intensive care unit prior to return to the operating room for definitive management of injuries and abdominal closure.[9-10] After splenectomy, patients should be vaccinated against pneumococcus, haemophilus, and meningococcus to reduce the risk of overwhelming postsplenectomy sepsis.

Of note, management of children and adolescents with solid-organ injury differs dramatically from management of adult patients with similar grade of injury. Even when high-grade injuries are present, solid-organ injuries are typically successfully managed nonoperatively in young people with serial abdominal examinations, serial hematocrit testing, bowel rest, and bed rest.[6]

Hollow Viscus Injury

Intestine

Hollow viscus injuries (15%) involve the jejunum, duodenum, colon, and stomach, in decreasing order of frequency.[5] Injuries can include bowel perforation or tearing, bowel wall hematoma, and mesenteric tears that may devascularize the bowel and result in progressive ischemia or necrosis. The diagnosis of intestinal injury can be challenging, as a patient's symptoms, such as nausea, pain, and malaise, may be mild, delayed, and nonspecific. Further, both ultrasound and CT scan procedures are less sensitive for intestinal injury compared to solid-organ injuries. Therefore, clinicians must have a high index of suspicion in patients with a direct blow to the abdomen, a deceleration mechanism (eg, seat-belt injury) issue, or a handlebar injury.[11] Physical examination findings include tachycardia and abdominal wall bruising (ie, seat-belt sign).[12-13] Symptoms may include abdominal pain, peritonitis, and bilious emesis. Radiologic imaging is often normal, but nonspecific indicators may include free fluid or mesenteric edema or stranding. Laboratory findings include elevated lipase, white blood cell count, or lactate. Operative intervention is indicated in patients with peritonitis or in patients with a high suspicion for injury based on the presence of the previously described factors.

Bladder

Up to 85% of the time, injury to the urinary bladder is most commonly associated with a blunt mechanism of injury, with motor vehicle collision being the predominant mechanism.[14] The bladder is located near the pelvic floor posterior to the pubic symphysis and anterior to the vagina in women and rectum in men, separated from these organs by the prevesical space of Retzius. The peritoneum covers the dome, which is most vulnerable to injury as it rises into the peritoneal cavity with distension. Up to 90% of patients with such injuries will have concomitant pelvic fractures. Injuries are classified as extraperitoneal (60%) or intraperitoneal (30%). Up to 10% of patients will have a combined injury.[15] Patients most commonly present with gross hematuria, along with lower abdominal pain. Intraperitoneal injuries that may be initially missed can present with ileus, inability to void, azotemia, acidosis, electrolyte imbalances, and peritonitis.

In the hemodynamically stable patient, diagnosis may be made with retrograde cystography using either plain film or CT scan. CT cystography is most commonly used today and involves filling the bladder with 300 cc of water-soluble contrast via a Foley catheter[16] (see Figure 12-4). Management of injury is based on location and complexity. Simple extraperitoneal injuries are managed using catheter drainage alone for 2 to 3 weeks, with cystography performed prior to removal. Complex extraperitoneal injuries, such as open pelvic fractures, concurrent rectal or vaginal injury, or bladder neck injury, often require surgical repair. Intraperitoneal injuries always warrant surgical repair, as these are often large, and leakage of urine risks sepsis and peritonitis.[17]

Appendicitis

The appendix is located at the inferior tip of the cecum, deriving its blood supply from the appendiceal branch of the ileocolic artery. It works to secrete immunoglobulins, particularly immunoglobulin A. Appendicitis—inflammation

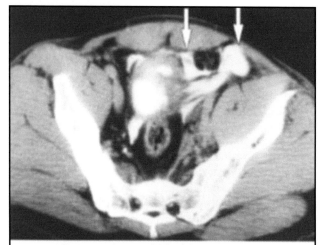

Intraperitoneal bladder rupture

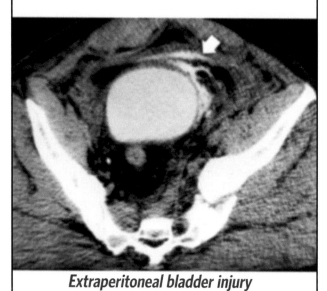

Extraperitoneal bladder injury

Figure 12-4. Intraperitoneal and extraperitoneal bladder rupture.

and infection of the appendix—has a lifetime occurrence of 7%, with one-third of all cases occurring in those below age 18 years. The highest incidence occurs in males age 10 to 14 and females age 15 to 19. The most common cause of appendicitis is mechanical obstruction with an appendicolith. Other causes include hyperplasia of lymphoid tissue and neoplasm.[18] Luminal obstruction results in progressive inflammation and pressure due to bacterial overgrowth and accumulation of secretions. The most commonly involved bacteria include *Escherichia coli* and *Bacteroides fragilis*. The distension of the appendix stretches visceral nerve fibers, resulting in the vague epigastric pain that is often the first sign of appendicitis. When inflammatory changes affect the serosa, there is extension to the parietal peritoneum, resulting in localized right lower quadrant pain.

Findings of appendicitis on examination depend on the location of the appendiceal tip. An anterior appendix will present with the classic point tenderness at McBurney's point, located one-third the distance from the anterior superior iliac spine along a direct line to the umbilicus. Rosving's sign—pain in the right lower quadrant when the left lower quadrant is palpated—is an indicator of localized peritoneal inflammation. A pelvic appendix is indicated by the obturator sign, elicited by passive internal rotation of the flexed right thigh. Finally, a retrocecal appendix is indicated by the psoas sign, elicited by positioning the patient on his or her left side and extending the right thigh, stretching the iliopsoas muscle, causing pain.[19]

In the pediatric population, ultrasound imaging is the modality of choice. A distended, noncompressible appendix, with a diameter of 6 mm or greater, indicates appendicitis (Figure 12-5). In the older adolescent or adult, CT scan is the modality of choice and may demonstrate a distended, thickened appendix with periappendiceal fluid or fat stranding.[20] Caution must be taken to not completely rely on imaging, as patients may have appendicitis without manifested imaging findings. Furthermore, particularly in very young persons other conditions, such as constipation, may mimic appendicitis. However, given the possible severe sequelae of missed diagnosis, an up-to-30% negative appendectomy rate has been accepted.

Management of appendicitis depends on clinical presentation. In the past, appendicitis was considered a surgical emergency. However, in current practice, appendectomy may be performed within 24 hours of presentation without change in morbidity or mortality after antibiotic treatment is initiated. In most patients, laparoscopic appendectomy is the procedure of choice. Compared to open appendectomy, this has been shown to have lower morbidity and shorter hospital length of stay. However, open appendectomy is still used for patients who present in extremis or in situations where laparoscopy is unsafe. Postoperative antibiotics are generally unnecessary unless a patient is found to have perforation during appendectomy, which may occur in up to 4% of cases.[21] In these instances, a 7-day course is often prescribed. For patients who are found to have a periappendiceal abscess at initial diagnosis, imaging-guided drain placement with a course of antibiotics is the initial management of choice, and patients are often discharged with outpatient follow-up to determine any need for interval appendectomy.[22] Postoperatively, patients are instructed to avoid heavy lifting or strenuous activity for at least 2 weeks, with gradual increase in activity as tolerated after this period.

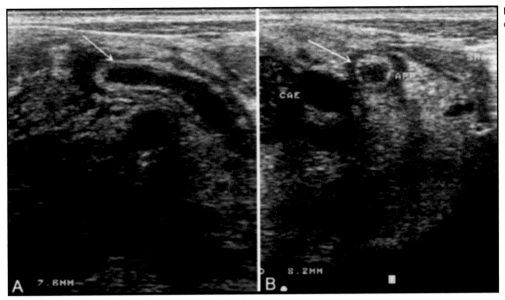

Figure 12-5. Ultrasound demonstrates acute appendicitis

CHAPTER SUMMARY

The evaluation of abdominal pain in the athlete can carry a broad differential diagnosis with a varying spectrum of presentation. Particularly in a population with high physiologic reserve, high clinical suspicion for significant injury is a necessity among training staff and medical professionals to ensure the administration of appropriate and timely care. For patients with suspected traumatic injury, particularly in contact sports, evaluation at a trauma center has been shown to improve outcomes, with decreased mortality and morbidity. A thorough history elicited from the patient, as well as witnesses to the injury, is critical, along with close attention to physical examination findings such as areas of ecchymosis, abrasions, and lacerations. When considering adjunct imaging, the desire to limit radiation exposure in the pediatric population should always be weighed against the consequences of a missed injury. This is particularly important in patients with a distracting injury. For example, patients presenting with femur fracture may have concomitant back or neck injury, but they may not be able to express pain symptoms in those areas, given the obvious extremity fracture.

In addition to traumatic injury, trainers and team medical personnel should be cognizant of other possible causes of pain and illness in the athlete. A collaborative communication between guardians and training staff can help ensure that symptoms are monitored—and the evolution of symptoms is monitored—and prompt medical attention is sought when necessary, as consequences of delayed or missed diagnosis in conditions such as appendicitis may be devastating.

High suspicion for illness and injury is necessary in the athlete, given the high physiologic reserve as well as the multitude of diagnoses that may impact these individuals.

Intervention at an appropriate specialty center, particularly in cases of trauma, greatly improves outcomes and return to the field.

CHAPTER REVIEW QUESTIONS

1. What is the most commonly injured solid organ in the body?
2. Define peritonitis.
3. What is meant by the phrase "damage-control surgery?"
4. What is the bowel mesentery, and what is the result of injury to this structure?
5. What are the 2 types of bladder injury?

ANSWERS

1. Spleen
2. Inflammation of the peritoneal lining of the abdomen, resulting in severe pain.
3. An initial operation conducted to control bleeding and gross contamination only with the intention of returning the patient to the operating room for definitive repair and closure following appropriate resuscitation and stabilization in an intensive care unit setting.
4. A double layer of parietal peritoneum attaching the intestines to the abdominal wall and serving as a conduit for vasculature, nerves, and lymphatics to the intestines. Injury often results in ischemia to the bowel due to concomitant injury to vasculature contained within.
5. Intraperitoneal and extraperitoneal.

REFERENCES

1. Osler TM, Vane DW, Tepas JJ, Rogers FB, Shackford SR, Badger GJ. Do pediatric trauma centers have better survival rates than adult trauma centers? An examination of the National Pediatric Trauma Registry. *J Trauma.* 2001;50(1):96-101.

2. Oyetunji TA, Haider AH, Downing SR, et al. Treatment outcomes of injured children at adult level 1 trauma centers: are there benefits from added specialized care? *Am J Surg.* 2011;201(4):445-449.

3. Potoka DA, Schall LC, Gardner MJ, Stafford PW, Peitzman AB, Ford HR. Impact of pediatric trauma centers on mortality in a statewide system. *J Trauma.* 2000;49(2):237-245.

4. Gutiérrez CE. Pediatric Trauma. In: Tintinalli JE, Stapczynski J, Ma O, Yealy DM, Meckler GD, Cline DM. eds. *Tintinalli's Emergency Medicine: A Comprehensive Study Guide, 8e.* New York, NY: McGraw-Hill; 2016. http://accessmedicine.mhmedical.com/content.aspx?bookid=1658&sectionid=109381281.

5. Keller MS. Blunt injury to solid abdominal organs. *Semin Pediatr Surg.* 2004;13(2):106-111.

6. Holmes JF, Lillis K, Monroe D, et al. Identifying children at very low risk of clinically important blunt abdominal injuries. *Ann Emerg Med.* 2013;62(2):107-162.

7. Notrica DM, Eubanks JW 3rd, Tuggle DW, et al. Nonoperative management of blunt liver and spleen injury in children: Evaluation of the ATOMAC guideline using GRADE. *J Trauma Acute Care Surg.* 2015;79(4):683-693.

8. Potoka DA, Gaines BA, Leppaniemi A, Peitzman AB. Management of blunt pancreatic trauma: what's new? *Eur J Trauma Emerg Surg.* 2015;41(3):239-250.

9. Richardson JD, Franklin GA, Lukan JK, et al. Evolution in the management of hepatic trauma: a 25-year perspective. *Ann Surg.* 2000;232(3):324-330.

10. Stylianos S. Abdominal packing for severe hemorrhage. *J Ped Surg.* 1998;33(2):339-342.

11. Sturm PF, Glass RB, Sivit CJ, Eichelberger MR. Lumbar compression fractures secondary to lap-belt use in children. *J Pediatr Orthop.* 1995;15(4):521-523.

12. Lutz N, Nance ML, Kallan MJ, Arbogast KB, Durbin DR, Winston FK.. Incidence and clinical significance of abdominal wall bruising in restrained children involved in motor vehicle crashes. *J Ped Surg.* 2004;39(6):972-975.

13. Paris C, Brindamour M, Ouimet A, St-Vil D. Predictive indicators for bowel injury in pediatric patients who present with a positive seat belt sign after motor vehicle collision. *J Ped Surg.* 2010;45(5):921-924.

14. Diebert CM, Spencer BA. The association between operative repair of bladder injury and improved survival: results from the National Trauma Data Bank. *J Urol.* 2011;186(1):151.

15. Gomez RG, Ceballos L, Coburn M, et al. Consensus statement on bladder injuries. *BJU Int.* 2004;94(1):27-32.

16. Quagliano PV, Delair SM, Malhotra AK. Diagnosis of blunt bladder injury: a prospective comparative study of computed tomography cystography and conventional retrograde cystography. *J Trauma.* 2006;61(2):410.

17. Wessells H. Genitourinary injuries. In: Peitzman AB, Rhodes M, Schwab CW, Yealy DM, Fabian TC, eds. *The Trauma Manual: Trauma and Acute Care Surgery.* 4th ed. Philadelphia, PA: Lippincott, Williams, and Wilkins; 2013:395-403.

18. Rabah R. Pathology of the appendix in children: an institutional experience and review of literature. *Pediatr Radiol.* 2007;37(1):15-20.

19. Bundy DG, Byerley JS, Liles EA. Does this child have appendicitis? *JAMA.* 2007;298(4):438.

20. Schuh S, Chan K, Langer JC, et al. Properties of serial ultrasound clinical diagnostic pathway in suspected appendicitis and related computed tomography use. *Acad Emerg Med.* 2015;22(4):406-414.

21. Simillis C, Symeonides P, Shorthouse AJ, Tekkis PP. A meta-analysis comparing conservative treatment versus acute appendectomy for complicated appendicitis (abscess or phlegmon). *Surgery.* 2010;147:818-829.

22. Peter SD, Aguayo P, Fraser JS, et al. Initial laparoscopic appendectomy versus initial nonoperative management and interval appendectomy for perforated appendicitis with abscess: a prospective, randomized trial. *J Pediatr Surg.* 2010;45:236-240.

13

Emergencies Related to Conditioning and Exercise

Sarah Manspeaker, PhD, LAT, ATC and Kelley Henderson, EdD, LAT, ATC

CHAPTER KEY WORDS

- Creatine kinase
- Exercise-associated hyponatremia
- Exertional rhabdomyolysis
- Hypohydration
- Myoglobinuria
- Sickle cell trait
- Sodium

CHAPTER SCENARIO

Martin, a Division I football player, traveled from his home university in Tampa, FL, (elevation: 48 feet) to Boulder, CO, (elevation: 5,328 feet) to play in a conference game. In the first half of the game, Martin reported to the athletic trainer with cramping in his left leg. He was treated with stretching exercises, given oral hydration products, and returned to the game. During the second quarter, Martin began to experience significant pain, rated 10/10, in his low back, as well as in his left side beneath his ribs, and shortness of breath. He was immediately removed from the game and transported to a local hospital for further evaluation. Throughout the evening at the hospital, Martin began to develop a fever, which topped out at 102°F. A complete blood count revealed elevated white blood cell count.

SCENARIO RESOLUTION

Following an abdominal computed tomography scan, Martin was diagnosed with a splenic infarct as a result of the decreased oxygen to the spleen at the high altitude. Martin was hospitalized for 5 days, and he was then released to fly back to Florida, with instructions for conservative treatment and rest until the spleen had healed. He did not participate in any activity for 3 weeks and began an acclimation protocol to return to full participation that took 3 weeks.

INTRODUCTION

The incidence of medical emergencies directly related to participation in conditioning and exercise is rare. When such emergencies occur, the associated conditions are characterized by the development of signs and symptoms often related to the timing, location, and intensity of the physical activity. Even though these conditions could be fatal, proper recognition and treatment can prevent sudden death in athletes.

Health care providers should be familiar with the signs and symptoms associated with conditions such as exercise-associated hyponatremia, exertional collapse associated with sickle cell trait, and exertional rhabdomyolysis. In addition, they should understand the contributing environmental and exercise intensity factors that may increase risk for development of such conditions. Being able to

Feld F., Gorse KM, Blanc RO
Non-Orthopedic Emergency Care in Athletics (pp 105-113).

quickly recognize signs and symptoms of these conditions should lead to decreased time to diagnosis, with subsequent increase in effective treatment methods, prevention of catastrophic outcomes, and ultimate return to activity. This chapter will present an overview of each of the mentioned conditions, the predisposing factors or causes of the conditions, the related signs and symptoms, and treatment and return to activity guidelines.

Exercise-Associated Hyponatremia

The body requires a delicate balance between fluid and electrolytes, particularly among individuals involved in physical activity.[1] Fluid intake before, during, and after exercise is important, given the concern about hypohydration[2]; however, it is possible to drink excessive amounts of fluid to become overhydrated. This overhydration results in more water than nutrients in the cells,[3,4] thus resulting in hyponatremia. During exercise, the fluid balance and subsequent increase in water rather than nutrients can be termed *exercise-associated hyponatremia* (EAH).

EAH is closely related to the amount of water present in the body. The terms *hypohydration*, or loss of body water, and *dehydration*, or deficit of body water caused by hypohydration, are important to understand in relation to the differences from EAH.[2] The condition of EAH refers not to body water content, but rather to the amounts of electrolytes, specifically sodium, present within the body. Hyponatremia is simply the decrease in blood sodium concentrate.[3] From a clinical standpoint, EAH occurs during or within 24 hours after physical activity and is marked by a serum, plasma, or blood sodium concentration less than 135 mmol/L (normal values range from 135 to 145 mmol/L).[3] It can be considered a potential medical emergency.[2]

Causes and Predisposing Factors

Several contributing factors may lead to the development of EAH. During exercise, these factors may include excessive fluid consumption, failure to excrete excess volume, and excessive sodium loss.[2,3] Furthermore, prolonged exercise may particularly influence the development of EAH. Each of these topics will be discussed further in this chapter.

Excessive fluid consumption, or overdrinking, is often accomplished when a person consumes more fluid than he or she can expel.[3,5] In simpler terms, a person drinks more fluid or water than is released through sweat and urine.[3] Timing of this ingestion typically matches periods of hydration and rehydration (eg, before or after physical activity). Sometimes, patients may show signs and symptoms of EAH (Table 13-1) but be diagnosed with hypohydration and given more water, thus increasing the likelihood for EAH. It is possible for someone to be both hypohydrated and hyponatremic.

In contrast to excessive fluid consumption, the lack of ability to excrete excess volume may also lead to EAH. For example, sweating is the primary mechanism for the body to dissipate heat.[5] The contents of sweat include water and electrolytes such as sodium, chloride, and potassium.[5] If a person does not sweat as much as he or she drinks water or other hypotonic fluids, the balance of nutrients in the body will decrease. This imbalance becomes even more pronounced during long periods of exercise as well as heat.[5] Specifically, these environmental factors have been linked to decreased blood flow and urine output, thus contributing to the development of EAH.[5]

Excessive sodium loss, which often occurs through sweating, may also lead to EAH.[3] Serum sodium levels are determined through the total content of exchangeable sodium and potassium in relation to body water.[3] When loss of these electrolytes occurs or when the amount of body water increases, hyponatremia results. For example, if a person sweats excessively, the nutrient balance may decrease significantly.[1,5] In athletics, this imbalance is often due to prolonged exercise, lack of acclimation to the environment, or inexperience in the activity being performed.[3,5] Additionally, general sodium content in the body may be decreased in those who have a low-sodium diet or those who do not consume drinks containing sodium.[5]

Prolonged exercise may be a direct contributor to the development of EAH. Physical activity lasting longer than 4 to 5 hours typically falls into this category.[3] During an event such as an ultramarathon or marathon, it is important to prevent both hypohydration and hyperhydration. Other participants who may be at risk for EAH are those who did not adequately train or who are inexperienced in the event, those with a slower running or performance pace, and individuals with a high or low body mass index.[1,3]

Signs and Symptoms

The signs and symptoms of EAH may vary, but they should always be considered by the athletic trainer. Some patients may be asymptomatic and not present with any significant signs or symptoms. As the sodium imbalance increases, symptoms may develop and can be categorized as either mild or severe. Mild EAH is often characterized by signs and symptoms of dizziness, lightheadedness, nausea, and/or weight gain.[3,5] More severe forms of EAH may present with the signs and symptoms of headache, nausea or vomiting, confusion or other change in mental status, dyspnea, or frothy sputum.[3,5] If left unrecognized or untreated, EAH may develop into a sequelae of seizure or coma, thus elevating the emergent nature of the patient's condition.[3] Table 13-1 provides an overview of the differential signs and symptoms between EAH and hypohydration.

Diagnostic Criteria

Diagnosis of EAH is best achieved through analysis of blood sodium concentrate. In the athletic training clinical setting, a finger stick and an express blood analyzer may

TABLE 13-1. DIFFERENTIATING EXERCISE-ASSOCIATED HYPONATREMIA FROM HYPOHYDRATION

	EXERCISE-ASSOCIATED HYPONATREMIA		HYPOHYDRATION
SIGNS	*Mild*	*Severe*	
Blood sodium levels	< 135 mmol/L	< 125 mmol/L	
Changes in mood/behavior	✓		
Muscle weakness or twitching	✓		
Apathy	✓		✓
Nausea/vomiting	✓	✓	
Diarrhea			✓
Weight gain	✓		
Frothy sputum		✓	
Weight loss			✓
Change in mental status	✓	✓	
Swelling of hands, feet, or both	✓		
SYMPTOMS	*Mild*	*Severe*	
Headache		✓	✓
Body chills			✓
Thirst			✓
Dyspnea		✓	✓
Dizziness/lightheadedness	✓		✓

Adapted from National Athletic Trainers' Association. Consensus statement: Sickle cell trait and the athlete. 2007. https://www.nata.org/sites/default/files/sicklecelltraitandtheathlete.pdf. Accessed September 28, 2018.

be used.[6] In the hospital setting, a physician may order an electrolyte panel or base metabolic panel to determine the levels of sodium present in the blood. From a combined diagnostic and clinical symptom standpoint, a blood sodium value of less than 135 mmol/L would elicit symptoms. Values below 125 mmol/L would warrant immediate administration of treatment to increase sodium levels; whereas patients with values less than 120 mmol/L of sodium would likely present in a comatose state and require advanced emergency medical attention.[3]

Treatment

Asymptomatic patients can transition to symptomatic if hypotonic fluids are ingested; therefore, it is of utmost importance to recognize and treat EAH early.[3] When identified, EAH should be treated on an individual basis to address the specific severity of presenting signs and symptoms.[7] While onsite at an event, a patient displaying mild EAH should be under observation for progression into a symptomatic stage. Hypotonic and isotonic fluids should be restricted until the patient is urinating freely. Treatment may consist of administration of either oral

hypertonic saline (HTS) such as concentrated bouillon or 3% to 5% sodium chloride (NaCl) with added flavoring, or intravenous HTS.[3] Those individuals presenting with severe EAH should receive immediate administration of intravenous (IV) HTS and be prepared for transport to the emergency department.[3] Clinical practice guidelines for treatment of EAH in the hospital setting have been established and should be based on severity of symptoms and the serum sodium values. Treatment guidelines include 3% NaCl administered intravenously over a 20-minute period, followed by a blood sodium retest. This treatment should be continued until there is a 5-mmol/L increase in serum sodium.[7]

Return to Activity

Currently, no consistent body of literature supports return-to-activity guidelines following treatment for EAH. When symptoms, including a normal serum sodium level, have resolved and the athlete has been cleared by a physician, he or she may begin to transition back to activity. There should be an individualized hydration plan developed as well as further education on excessive fluid intake.

Prevention

Prevention of EAH begins with education regarding drinking behaviors and monitoring hydration through body weight. Athletes, parents, coaches, and event support crews need to understand the dangers of overdrinking. The thirst sensation can prevent excess dehydration while also preventing the excessive fluid intake contributing to the development of EAH. Individuals should be educated on the importance of not drinking in excess of sweat rate. If an athlete secretes salty sweat and will be involved in events lasting longer than 4 to 6 hours, he or she may consider consuming food or drinks containing sodium.[5] Although sodium supplementation equal to fluid loss may be beneficial, it will not prevent EAH if there is excessive fluid intake.[3,8] Due to the wide variety of sweat rates and renal excretion capacity, specific guidelines for fluid consumption should be individualized.[3,5] For event management and support teams, it may be beneficial to decrease the number of fluid stations as well as provide appropriate drinking advice to event participants.[3] Educational programs for athletes, parents, coaches, and onsite medical staff should also include recognition of signs and symptoms of EAH, management of EAH, and the immediate need for medical attention if EAH is suspected.[3]

Sickle Cell Trait

Sickle cell trait (SCT) is a hereditary condition in which the red blood cells of the body are not uniform. Specifically, one hemoglobin gene (A) is shaped normally, and the other hemoglobin gene (S) is abnormally shaped.[9] An estimated more than 4-million people in the United States have SCT. In general, most people identified as carrying the SCT have no adverse health effects due to the trait.[10,13] For people with SCT, the abnormal shape of the red blood cells decreases the ability to carry oxygen through the blood to the rest of the body.[9,11] If this oxygen delivery is impaired for a period of time, life-threatening impacts on the body may occur.

Sickle cell abnormalities are identified most often in people who have connections to locations where malaria is prevalent. The ethnicities associated with SCT may be traced to ancestry in areas such as Africa, South/Central America, Mediterranean countries, Hispanic countries, south Asian countries, Middle Eastern areas, and the Caribbean.[12] People who carry the SCT do not necessarily have sickle cell anemia, and the SCT cannot turn into sickle cell disease. To have sickle cell disease, a person must have 2 abnormal hemoglobin genes.[13]

Of primary concern to the athletic trainer is exercise collapse associated with SCT (ECAST).[14,15] During exercise or exertion, the abnormal hemoglobin may change from a round shape to more of a quarter-moon shape, known as *sickling*. This is a medical emergency called *exertional sickling*, and it poses a significant risk to athletes, as it may result in sudden death.[14,15] SCT has also been identified as a potential contributor to the development of exertional rhabdomyolysis, which will be presented later in the chapter.

Another potential complication associated with SCT and activity is impact on the spleen. The spleen is one of the most-often affected organs in SCT carriers, and complications may result in splenomegaly.[16] Clinicians should be aware of the potential for splenomegaly and potential complications, such as rupture, during activity. Complications due to splenic enlargement have direct associations with increased morbidity of SCT and may, in some cases, lead to mortality.[16]

Causes and Predisposing Factors

During exercise or exertion, the oxygen carrying abilities of the blood may be decreased due to the resultant S-shape of the abnormal hemoglobin.[9] Specifically, these sickled red blood cells may build up and block normal blood flow to muscle and other tissue.[15] It has been theorized that there may be a quick increase in epinephrine during exercise that could contribute to the sickled red blood cells becoming sticky, thus further cutting off blood flow to muscles.[15]

Athletes who carry the SCT may be at increased risk of developing ECAST based on their environment, hydration level, and presence of asthma.[9,13,17] Environmental factors include high heat, high humidity, and high altitude. High heat and humidity influence the body's ability to maintain hydration levels. Hydration is an important consideration for proper athletic performance. Altitude is of significant note, as the higher the elevation, the less oxygen is available. Due to the decreased ability of red blood cells to carry oxygen when sickled, the already-decreased oxygen levels at high altitude can further decrease the body's ability to circulate the much-needed oxygen. Sickling events may often be seen in athletes who have participated in maximal exertion exercise over a short time frame, such as a few minutes.[9,13,17]

Signs and Symptoms of Exercise Collapse Associated With Sickle Cell Trait

For athletes experiencing a sickling event, several signs and symptoms may occur. Initially, the patient will present with muscle pain, cramping, and weakness, particularly in the lower extremity and back.[13,17,18] Further evaluation will likely reveal that the muscle weakness is greater than pain, and the muscles feel normal upon palpation. Many athletes have been noted to slump to the ground during a sickling event or report that they cannot go any further, and just stop activity.[13,18] Additional signs may include shortness of breath during or immediately following exercise, as well as fatigue and difficulty recovering after exertion.[17,19] In many cases, this clinical presentation may warrant a differential diagnosis with heat illness and/or cardiac conditions.[13] In comparison to these conditions, the patient

TABLE 13-2. TELLTALE FEATURES AMONG COMMON NON-TRAUMA CAUSES OF ON-FIELD COLLAPSE

SICKLING	CARDIAC	HEAT STROKE	ASTHMA
Weakness > pain	No cramping	Fuzzy thinking	Usually known asthma
Slumps to ground	Falls suddenly	Bizarre behavior	Prior episodes, poor control
Can talk at first	Unconscious	Incoherent	Breathless, may wheeze or not
Muscles "normal"	Limp or seizing	Can be in coma	Gasping, panicky, on hands/knees
Temperature < 103° F	Temperature irrelevant	Temperature often > 106° F	Auscultate: moving little air
Can occur early	No warning	Usually occurs late	Usually occurs after sprinting

Reprinted with permission from Eichner, ER. Sickle Cell Trait in Sport. *Curr Sports Med Rep.* 2010; 9(6): 347-351. © 2010 Wolters Kluwer

will often be able to communicate clearly, at least at first, and will have a rectal temperature below 103°F.[18] Not all patients will present the same. Some will have leg and low back symptoms, whereas others will have chest tightness. It is all individualized[18] (Table 13-2).

Diagnostic Criteria

Diagnosis of SCT typically occurs shortly after birth, as all babies are screened for the red blood cell anomaly of hemoglobin S. The screening may be performed for an adult as well. The National Collegiate Athletic Association recommends that athletic departments confirm SCT status for all student-athletes, either through birth record or evidence of recent screening. Students may elect to abstain from this screening but must sign a written release to do so. This requirement is somewhat controversial, as the American Society for Hematology (ASH) does not support this testing or disclosure of SCT status prior to athletic participation. Current ASH policies cite a lack of sufficient scientific evidence to support this requirement. Although ASH does support safe sports participation by those with SCT, it also supports voluntary screening, with the ability to obtain comprehensive counseling on the condition.[20]

Regarding diagnosis of the emergency condition ECAST, athletes typically present following a period of exercise at or near maximal exertion.[13] This maximal exertion effort may be for either a short time frame, such as repeat sprints, or activity of longer duration. No specific laboratory or clinical test confirms an on-field sickling event.[18]

Treatment

Swift recognition and management of ECAST is imperative to prevent catastrophic outcomes. During an on-field assessment, the clinician should determine the athlete's vital signs and continue to monitor. Early administration of

high-flow oxygen at a rate of 15 L/min with a nonrebreather mask is considered a good course of early treatment.[17,19] Patients should be immediately removed from activity, and hydration tactics should be initiated. Fast referral to the emergency department and activation of the emergency action plan and standard operating procedures should occur.

Treatment in the emergency department is similar to that of other emergent conditions identified in this text. Prior to arrival at the emergency department, it may be beneficial to inform the staff that the patient may have ECAST to ensure appropriate treatment is performed to prevent specific complications due to rhabdomyolysis.[18] Specifically, emphasis should be placed on aggressive fluid replacement, electrolyte administration, monitoring of blood gases, and assessment of cardiac vitals, including potential arrhythmias.[13]

Return to Activity

No evidence-based guidelines exist for return to activity following an ECAST event. Medical personnel should consider potential return when the patient is asymptomatic at rest and all organ function tests appear normal. This determination should be made as part of the interprofessional health care team in consideration of findings from the physician, athletic trainer, and all other members of the interdisciplinary team. Activity should be approached in a graded manner, with light exercise slowly progressing to increased levels of intensity over time. A patient returning to activity after ECAST should also receive further education about physical activity, intensity levels, and the role of hydration, heat, and altitude.[13]

Prevention

Although the occurrence of ECAST should be rare, steps may be taken to decrease the risk of an event. ASH recommends patient education and implementation of universal preventive measures similar to those used for the prevention of heat illness; which include heat acclimation, appropriate ratios for work-to-rest, thorough hydration, and nutrition.[20] Furthermore, ensuring that medical staff members are available and able to recognize ECAST early and provide appropriate treatment upon such recognition drastically decreases the chance of death.

The patient, family, coaches, and any other members of the interprofessional health care team should receive information regarding SCT and participation in athletics. The team should review and watch for signs and symptoms of ECAST. Because it is not the condition of SCT itself that causes an issue, the role of hydration, acclimatization, and the environment should be shared in detail.[21]

For environmental conditions, proper acclimatization for the associated sport should occur according to best practice recommendations by sport. Athletes with SCT should be able to set their own conditioning pace, as well as be allotted extended rest periods between bouts. It may be considered that SCT carriers be excluded from timed performance activities, such as repeat sprints, stair-climbing workouts, and mile runs for performance time.[19,22] Standard precautions for participation in heat and humid environments should also be instructed and monitored during participation.[22] From a nutritional standpoint, these athletes should avoid energy drinks that contain high amounts of caffeine or other products that may contribute to dehydration. As with most athletic participation, revisions during periods of illness, including perhaps withdrawing from athletic activity when sick, should be considered.

Because altitude has a direct impact on oxygen availability to the body, athletes with SCT should consider the risk-to-reward ratio for participation in high altitudes. If such participation is anticipated, it will be necessary to dedicate ample time to modify training by decreasing intensity and length of activity, especially early in arrival to the high-altitude area. During these times of participation, it will be necessary to have supplemental oxygen available.[19]

Exertional Rhabdomyolysis

Rhabdomyolysis occurs when muscle tissue, specifically skeletal muscle, breaks down, and the contents cross the cell membrane and flow within the bloodstream.[23] This condition occurs most often during events such as car accidents, crush injuries, drug overdoses, and infections.[23] Among the active population, intense exercise may lead to excessive muscle breakdown and subsequent release of contents into the bloodstream. This is termed *exertional rhabdomyolysis (ER)*.[24]

Incidence of ER has been reported at a rate of nearly 26,000 people per year[25]; however, accurate estimates in the general population are difficult to determine due to undiagnosed or late presentation of symptoms.[26] ER has been reported most often in the military population due to the intense nature of training activities, but the number of reported cases among athletes has been increasing.[27,28]

The primary muscle cell contents of concern during ER include creatine kinase (CK), myoglobin, calcium, and other minerals and acids.[29] The presence of CK and myoglobin in the blood places significant stress on the kidneys that may result in a sequelae of acute renal failure and/or cardiac arrhythmias that could lead to death.[29]

Causes and Predisposing Factors

For those participating in athletics, exercise of extreme intensity has been linked to the development of ER. Often, those diagnosed with ER report recent performance of physical activity at a higher intensity level than what they typically do, with most cases occurring during preseason activity or after periods of rest, such as a holiday break.[27] Aspects of the activity most often increase in relation to length of time, number of repetitions, focus on a specific muscle group, and/or emphasis on eccentric muscle contractions.[30] Other factors that have been linked to potential development of ER include medication and drug use, environmental factors, and carrying the SCT.[31] In consideration of earlier chapter topics, ER may occur in the presence of hyponatremia[32] or hyperthermia.[26]

Signs and Symptoms

Patients with ER typically report initial signs and symptoms within 24 to 48 hours following the associated workout.[33] Specifically, the patient's history will reveal a recent bout of intense or strenuous exercise, often including repeated eccentric contractions or repetitive exercises.[33,34] An early sign includes significant muscle pain much greater than that of delayed-onset muscle soreness in the muscle group of focus; it may or may not include associated weakness, stiffness, and swelling.[23] Patients may report cola- or tea-colored urine, which could indicate myoglobinuria.[23]

Diagnostic Criteria

Although a conclusive set of criteria for diagnosis of ER has not been established, most clinicians agree that serum CK, myoglobinuria, and electrolyte levels should be obtained to contribute to the potential diagnosis. Normal CK values typically range from 20 to 200 IU/L and will often be elevated in excess of 5% to 10% during an ER event.[35] Myoglobinuria values may increase beyond the normal level of 15 mg/L, although this finding is not always present in patients with ER.[35,36] Establishment of these values should occur in the hospital setting via blood test; therefore, early recognition and referral to the emergency department is key.

CK levels are not typically included as part of baseline assessment for those participating in athletics and, as such, it is difficult to use this value as a universal indicator of ER. These CK values may vary based on the person's gender, race, and physical conditioning status.[37] In regard to differential diagnosis, the CK level would be of pertinent value in differentiating ECAST from ER in that ECAST does not typically result in increased CK levels.[38]

Treatment

Treatment of ER typically commences when blood tests indicate CK levels between 10,000 and 20,000 IU/L.[37] When ER is determined, fluid replacement or resuscitation via IV saline fluids should be administered quickly. Administration of these IV fluids may include the addition of compounds such as sodium chloride or potassium chloride, though evidence support of these additions varies.[27] Treatment with IV fluids should occur at a rate of 200 to 1000 mL/hour, with an aim to preserve renal function.[39,40] While the amount of fluids delivered will vary, urinary output should be monitored and maintained between 200 and 300 mL/hour until myoglobinuria, if present, has resolved. Typically, the patient will be hospitalized for the duration of this treatment and withheld from all physical activity until blood tests have returned to normal ranges and all signs and symptoms have resolved.

Patients who are known to have SCT and who are diagnosed with ER may require more aggressive fluid resuscitation and closer monitoring of renal function. Due to the impact that sickling has on blood flow to the organs, these patients are at greater risk for kidney failure and may require hemodialysis.[27,41]

Return to Activity

Prior to any physical activity, the patient should be asymptomatic, with a normal physical examination, have CK levels near 5000 IU/L, and receive clearance from a physician.[42,43] The factors of time to recovery, history of the individual and family, and symptoms of ER should be considered when determining the appropriate path to return to activity. Based on these factors, the patient should be classified into a category of either suspicion of high risk of recurrence of ER or lower risk for recurrence of ER. If the patient is at a higher risk, then further physician evaluation is warranted. If the patient is classified as lower risk, then a 3-phase approach including environmental considerations and activity level can begin.[30,44] These phases of activity should be gradual, individualized, and emphasize aquatic therapy. Each phase should include monitoring of symptoms via urinalysis and serum CK levels prior to transitioning to the next phase.

Prevention

One of the most significant considerations for ER is how to prevent the condition from developing. Any person with

a role in physical activity, from coaches to athletes to athletic trainers to strength and conditioning personnel, should be aware of how ER develops and the appropriate decisions for activity to prevent its occurrence. Specific aspects to address should include the heat and humidity levels, the amount of repetition and intensity of the activity, and the time period of the workout in relation to competition season.[27,45] In general, each of these factors should be kept to a minimum, allowing for a graded, individualized level of conditioning prior to the introduction of more strenuous exercise. Personnel should avoid sudden increases in training volume and be aware of repetitive, strenuous loads that overly tax one specific muscle group. For athletes known to have SCT, all previously outlined preventive measures should be enforced to avoid development of ER.

CHAPTER SUMMARY

Although rare, medical emergencies directly related to participation in exercise and physical activity may occur. The conditions presented in this chapter may occur at any time; therefore, it is important for health care providers to remain aware and monitor participants during all activities so they can recognize changes in performance level and/or development of signs and symptoms early. The cause, presentation, prehospital care, and diagnostic procedures for these conditions vary, and although these aspects are different, the return to activity is somewhat similar in that resolution of all signs and symptoms, combined with a gradual return to activity, are recommended. Remaining knowledgeable in best practices for these conditions could help to decrease the chance of catastrophic outcomes during athletic participation.

CHAPTER REVIEW QUESTIONS

1. Discuss with a classmate or clinical supervisor why athletes with SCT may experience difficulty in performing at high altitudes.
2. What specific recommendations would you make to your coaches and members of the field hockey team regarding sodium intake and hydration during the first week of preseason training?
3. What diagnostic processes are required to achieve diagnosis of exertional collapse associated with SCT?
4. What are the laboratory tests and applicable diagnostic threshold values associated with exercise-related hyponatremia, ECAST, and exertional rhabdomyolysis?
5. In a small group, discuss how your emergency action plan would be different for the conditions of exercise-related hyponatremia, ECAST, and exertional rhabdomyolysis.

ANSWERS

1. Altitude is of significant note as the higher the elevation, the less oxygen is available. Due to the decreased ability of red blood cells to carry oxygen when sickled, the already-decreased oxygen levels at high altitude can further decrease the body's ability to circulate the much-needed oxygen.

2. I would recommend that all players ingest an increased amount of sodium to replace the amounts lost during activity. Given the necessary balance between sodium and water, ingesting too much water in comparison to sodium will deplete stores of sodium (and other electrolytes) in the body. During the first week of preseason training, given the increased demands of physical activity and often a hot environment, it is appropriate to increase sodium intake through beverages containing sodium, rather than relying solely on water as a hydration mechanism.

3. There is no specific test for ECAST. A thorough history, including determination of a positive blood test for SCT, history of exercise at or near maximal exertion, muscle pain, cramping and weakness, shortness of breath, and potential slumping to the ground, would be needed to arrive at this diagnosis.

4. EAH—blood sodium levels below 135 mmol/L
   a. ECAST—positive for SCT based on a blood test and signs or symptoms following exercise at or near maximal exertion
   b. ER—CK levels above 200 IU/L

5. Although each of these conditions is emergent in nature and will require activation of the emergency action plan, each has unique requirements for initial treatment during the emergency. During an EAH event, the patient will need to be given oral HTS or IV HTS. In the emergency department, a blood test will need to be administered to determine blood sodium levels. During emergency treatment of ECAST, early administration of high-flow oxygen is warranted. For ER, fast recognition of signs and symptoms, with subsequent referral to ED for testing and fluid resuscitation, would be required.

REFERENCES

1. Rodriguez NR. Position of the American Dietetic Association, Dietitians of Canada, and the American College of Sports Medicine: nutrition and athletic performance. *J Am Diet Assoc.* 2009;109(3):709-731.
2. McDermott BP, Anderson SA, Armstrong LE, et al. National Athletic Trainers' Association position statement: fluid replacement for the physically active. *J Athl Train.* 2017;52(9):877-895.
3. Hew-Butler T, Rosner MH, Fowkes-Godek S, et al. Statement of the third international exercise-associated hyponatremia consensus development conference, Carlsbad, California, 2015. *Clin J Sport Med.* 2015;25:303-320.
4. Noakes TD. Is drinking to thirst optimum? *Ann Nutr Metab.* 2010;57(suppl 2):9-17.
5. Montain SJ. Strategies to prevent hyponatremia during prolonged exercise. *Curr Sports Med Rep.* 2008;7(4):S28-S35.
6. Mohseni M, Silvers S, McNeil R, et al. Prevalence of hyponatremia, renal dysfunction, and other electrolyte abnormalities among runners before and after completing a marathon or half marathon. *Sports Health.* 2011;3(2):145-151.
7. Spasovski G, Vanholder R, Allolio B, et al. Clinical practice guidelines on the diagnosis and treatment of hyponatremia. *NDT Plus.* 2014;29(suppl 2):i1-139.
8. Hoffman MD, Stuempfle KJ. Sodium supplementation and exercise-associated hyponatremia during prolonged exercise. *Med Sci Sport Ex.* 2015;47(9):1782-1787.
9. Eichner ER. Sickle cell trait. *J Sport Rehab.* 2007;16:197-203.
10. Cleary MA. Sickle cell trait and exertional rhabdomyolysis. *Athl Ther Today.* 2003;8(5):66-67.
11. Jones JD, Kleiner DM. Awareness and identification of athletes with sickle cell disorders at historically black colleges and universities. *J Athl Train.* 1996;31:220-222.
12. Tsaras G, Owusu-Ansah A, Boateng FO, Amoateng-Adjepong Y. Complications associated with sickle cell trait: a brief narrative review. *Am J Med.* 2009;122:507-512.
13. O'Connor FG, Bergeron MF, Cantrell J, et al. ACSM and CHAMP summit on sickle cell trait: mitigating risks for warfighters and athletes. *Med Sci. Sports Exerc.* 2012;44:2045-2056.
14. Katch RK, Scarneo SE, Adams WM, et al. Top 10 research questions related to preventing sudden death in sport and physical activity. *Res Q Exerc Sport.* 2017;88(3):251-268.
15. Quattrone RD, Eichner ER, Beutler A, Adams WB, O'Connor FG. Exercise collapse associated with sickle cell trait (ECAST): case report and literature review. *Curr Sports Med Rep.* 2015;14(2):110-116.
16. Al-Salem AH. Splenic complications of sickle cell anemia and the role of splenectomy. *ISRN Hemtol.* 2011;864257. doi:10.5402/2011/864257.
17. Casa DJ, Almquist J, Anderson SA, et al. Sudden death in secondary school athletics programs: best practice recommendations. *J Athl Train.* 2013;48(4):546-553.
18. Eichner ER. Sickle cell trait in sport. *Curr Sports Med Rep.* 2010;9(6):347-351.
19. Casa DJ, Guskiewicz KM, Anderson SA, et al. National Athletic Trainers' Association position statement: preventing sudden death in sports. *J Athl Train.* 2012;47(1):96-118.

20. American Society of Hematology. Statement on screening for sickle cell trait and athletic participation. http://www.hematology.org/Advocacy/Statements/2650.aspx. Accessed September 21, 2018.

21. Sickle Cell Trait. NCAA.org - The Official Site of the NCAA. https://www.ncaa.org/sport-science-institute/sickle-cell-trait. Published September 12, 2016. Accessed September 28, 2018.

22. O'Connor DP, Fincher AL. Clinical pathology for athletic trainers: *Recognizing systemic disease.* 3rd ed. SLACK Incorporated; Thorofare, NJ: 2015.

23. Chatzizisis YS, Gesthimani M, Hatzitolios AI, Giannoglou GD. The syndrome of rhabdomyolysis: complications and treatment. *Eur J Intern Med.* 2008;19:568-574.

24. Baxter RE, Moore JH. Diagnosis and treatment of acute exertional rhabdomyolysis. *J Orthop Sports Phys Ther.* 2003;33(3):104-108.

25. Graves EJ, Gillum BS. Detailed diagnoses and procedures, National Hospital Discharge Survey, 1995. *Vital Health Stat.* 1997;13(130): 1-146.

26. Furman J. When exercise causes exertional rhabdomyolysis. *JAAPA.* 2015;28(4):38-43.

27. Manspeaker SA, Henderson KD, Riddle JD. Treatment of exertional rhabdomyolysis in athletes: a systematic review. *JBI Database System Rev Implement Rep.* 2016;14(6):117–147. doi:10.11124/JBISRIR-2016-001879.

28. O'Connor FG, Brennan FH, Campbell W, Heled Y, Deuster P. Return to physical activity after exertional rhabdomyolysis. *Curr Sports Med Rep.* 2008;(6):328-331.

29. Clarkson PM. Exertional rhabdomyolysis and acute renal failure in marathon runners. *Sports Med.* 2007;37(4.5):361-363.

30. Knapnick JJ, O'Connor FG. Exertional rhabdomyolysis: epidemiology, diagnosis, treatment, and prevention. *J Spec Oper Med.* 2016;16(3):65-71.

31. Rawson ES, Clarkson PM, Tarnopolsky MA. Perspectives on exertional rhabdomyolysis. *Sports Med.* 2017;47(suppl 1):S33-S49.

32. Cleary MA. Creatine kinase, exertional rhabdomyolysis and exercise-associated hyponatremia in ultra-endurance athletes: a critically appraised topic. *IJATT.* 2016;21(6):13-15.

33. Clarkson PM, Kearns AK, Rouzier P, Rubin R, Thompson PD. Serum creatine kinase levels and renal function measures in exertional muscle damage. *Med Sci Sports Exerc.* 2006;38(4):623-627.

34. Clarkson PM, Eichner ER. Exertional rhabdomyolysis: does elevated blood creatine kinase foretell renal failure? *Curr Sports Med Rep.* 2006;5:57-60.

35. Moghadam S, Oddis CV, Addarwal R. Approach to asymptomatic creatine kinase elevation. *Cleve Clin J Med.* 2016;83(1):37-42.

36. Bosch X, Poch E, Grau JM. Rhabdomyolysis and acute kidney injury. *N Engl J Med.* 2009;361:62-72.

37. Landau ME, Kenney K, Deuster P, Campbell W. Exertional rhabdomyolysis: a clinical review with a focus on genetic influences. *J Clin Neuromuscul Dis.* 2012;13:122-136.

38. Estes NAM, Link MS. Preparticipation athletic screening including an electrocardiogram: an unproven strategy for the prevention of sudden cardiac death in the athlete. *Pro Cardiovasc Dis.* 2012;54:451-454.

39. Harriston S. A review of rhabdomyolysis. *Dimens Crit Care Nurs.* 2004; 23(4):155-161.

40. Sauret JM, Marinides G, Wang GK. Rhabdomyolysis. *Am Fam Physician.* 2002;65:907-912.

41. Shelmadine BD, Baltensperger A, Wilson RL, Bowden RG. Rhabdomyolysis and acute renal failure in a sickle cell trait athlete: a case study. *Clin J Sport Med.* 2013;23:235-237.

42. Eichner ER. Exertional rhabdomyolysis. *Curr Sports Med Rep.* 2008;7(1):3-4.

43. Cleary MA, Ruiz D, Eberman L, Mitchell I, Binkley, H. Dehydration, cramping, and exertional rhabdomyolysis: a case report with suggestions for recover. *J Sport Rehabil.* 2007;16:244-259.

44. Asplund CA, O'Connor FG. Challenging return to play decisions: heat stroke, exertional rhabdomyolysis, and exertional collapse associated with sickle cell trait. *Sports Health.* 2016;8(2):117-125.

45. Sport Science Institute. NCAA.org - The Official Site of the NCAA. http://www.ncaa.org/health-and-safety/medical-conditions/ten-factors-can-increase-risk-exertional-rhabdomyolysis. Accessed April 4, 2019.

46. National Athletic Trainers' Association. Consensus statement: Sickle cell trait and the athlete. 2007. https://www.nata.org/sites/default/files/sicklecelltraitandtheathlete.pdf. Accessed September 28, 2018.

Appendix 1: Diabetic Athlete Treatment Algorithm

Feld F., Gorse KM, Blanc RO
Non-Orthopedic Emergency Care in Athletics (*pp* 115-116).
© 2020 Taylor & Francis Group.

Diabetic Athlete Treatment Algorithm

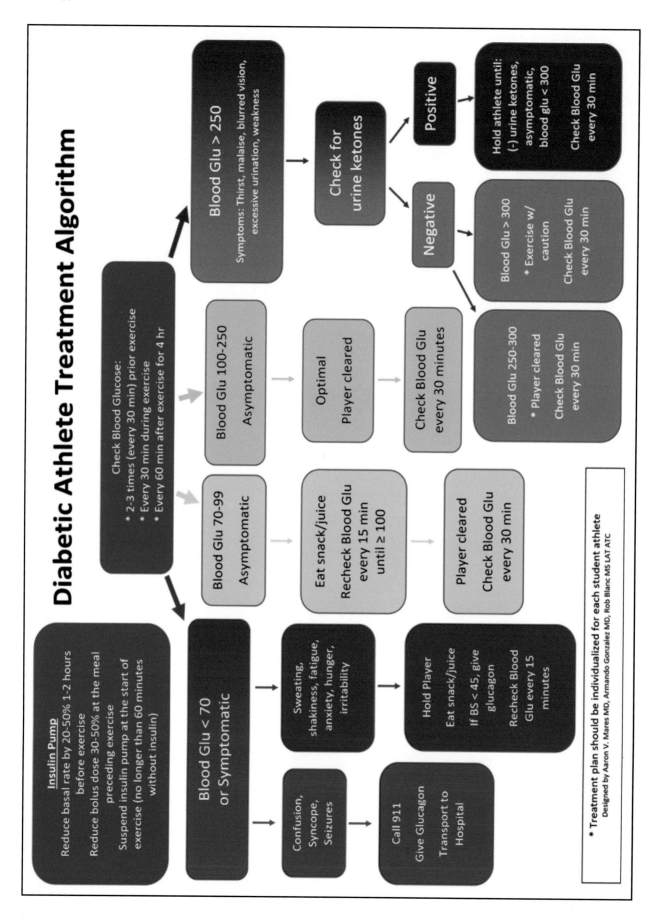

Insulin Pump

Reduce basal rate by 20-50% 1-2 hours before exercise

Reduce bolus dose 30-50% at the meal preceding exercise

Suspend insulin pump at the start of exercise (no longer than 60 minutes without insulin)

Check Blood Glucose:
* 2-3 times (every 30 min) prior exercise
* Every 30 min during exercise
* Every 60 min after exercise for 4 hr

Blood Glu > 250

Symptoms: Thirst, malaise, blurred vision, excessive urination, weakness

Check for urine ketones

Positive → Hold athlete until: (-) urine ketones, asymptomatic, blood glu <300

Check Blood Glu every 30 min

Negative → Blood Glu > 300
* Exercise w/ caution
Check Blood Glu every 30 min

Blood Glu 250-300
* Player cleared
Check Blood Glu every 30 min

Blood Glu 100-250

Asymptomatic → Optimal Player cleared → Check Blood Glu every 30 minutes

Blood Glu 70-99

Asymptomatic → Eat snack/juice Recheck Blood Glu every 15 min until ≥100 → Player cleared Check Blood Glu every 30 min

Blood Glu <70 or Symptomatic

Sweating, shakiness, fatigue, anxiety, hunger, irritability → Hold Player Eat snack/juice If BS < 45, give glucagon Recheck Blood Glu every 15 minutes

Confusion, Syncope, Seizures → Call 911 Give Glucagon Transport to Hospital

* Treatment plan should be individualized for each student athlete
Designed by Aaron V. Mares MD, Armando Gonzalez MD, Rob Blanc MS LAT ATC

Appendix 2: Intraveneous and Interosseous Access

Intravenous (IV) access has been mentioned frequently in the text for fluid resuscitation and medication administration. While this skill is not within the scope of practice for all health care professionals, everyone involved with athletic medicine should be aware of the intricacies of this intervention.

IV catheters are usually inserted into veins in the hands or arms, although the saphenous vein in the distal lower leg is an option if veins in the arms are not readily apparent.

Poiseuille's Law dictates the amount of fluid that can be infused.

Q	Flow rate
P	Pressure
r	Radius
η	Fluid viscosity
l	Length of tubing

$$Q = \frac{\pi P r^4}{8 \eta l}$$

Because the radius of the catheter to the fourth power is the most important factor in the equation, the larger the catheter used, the faster the fluid will infuse. A 14-gauge (g) catheter is the largest commonly used, whereas a 24-g is the smallest.

Catheter Size (gauge)	Length
14	1.16
16	1.16
20	1.0
22 (Pediatric size)	1.0
24 (Pediatric size)	1.0

Longer catheters are available, but although they are more stable, they also require more skill to insert and will slow fluid rates. The intern's vein near the anatomical snuffbox along the distal radius is a commonly accessed vein and will easily accept a 16-g large bore catheter. Veins on the dorsal aspect of the hand are considered more uncomfortable than other veins. Veins at the antecubital fossa will accept 14- to 16-g large bore catheters, but infiltration is more difficult to recognize, so these veins should be used with caution. If IV access is initiated for fluid administration with the intent to return the athlete to competition, the provider must remember that the large-bore IVs will require considerable time and pressure to occlude the site from bleeding after the catheter is discontinued. For this reason, an 18-g catheter should be the mainstay IV used in the athletic medicine arena.

Interosseous (IO) access is an option that should be reserved for critically injured athletes when peripheral IV access is problematic. A battery-powered drill is used to insert a metal 15-g needle into the intramedullary canal of

Feld F., Gorse KM, Blanc RO
Non-Orthopedic Emergency Care in Athletics (pp 117-118).
© 2020 Taylor & Francis Group.

the proximal medial tibia or the humeral head. Flow rates are equal to IV catheters, although rapid infusion of fluids through IOs is very painful. There is no literature to either support or refute the use of IO access in athletics regarding return to play. Many consider IO access easier than IV in patients who have collapsed veins secondary to cardiovascular dysfunction.

The most commonly used fluids for volume resuscitation are lactated ringers and normal saline. Each has advantages and disadvantages, so the team physician should decide which fluids will be used. Fluids containing dextrose are avoided in volume resuscitation.

Appendix 3: Bleed Bags

The Stop the Bleed campaign is a federal initiative that arose from the Hartford Consensus, and it is described in Chapters 2 and 9.

Every athletic venue should have a bleed bag available, not only for athletic injuries, but also for injuries to spectators and officials. Some items are mandatory, whereas others are optional, and the exact contents should be based on venue size and risk factors associated with the sport. Local emergency medical services should be consulted for input on the composition of bleed bags as well as possible provision of some items and training in their use.

MANDATORY ITEMS

- Tourniquets
  - Combat Application Tourniquet, Rapid Application Tourniquet System, and Stretch Wrap and Tuck Tourniquet
- Hemostatic gauze
  - Combat gauze
- Hemorrhage control bandage
  - Israeli combat dressing
- Cardiopulmonary resuscitation pocket mask
- Trauma shears
- Nitrile gloves
- Army battle dressings
  - Army battle dressing pads
- Sterile 4x4 gauze pads
- Kling dressing
  - 3- or 4-inch
- Adhesive tape
- Emergency blanket
- Chest seal dressing

Feld F., Gorse KM, Blanc RO
Non-Orthopedic Emergency Care in Athletics (pp 119-120).
© 2020 Taylor & Francis Group.

OPTIONAL ITEMS

- ACE wraps (3M)
- Skin stapler
- Skin closure glue
- Sterile gloves
- Leatherman's tool
- Forcible entry tool
- Chest needle decompression kit
  - Long 14g IV catheter with stopcock
- Small pulse oximeter unit
- Alcohol swabs
- Steri-Strip (Nexcare) or butterfly closures

Appendix 4: Individualized Seizure Response Plan

MY SEIZURE RESPONSE PLAN

Name: _____

Birth Date: _____

Address: _____

Phone: _____

1st Emergency Contact/Relation: _____

Phone: _____

2nd Emergency Contact/Relation: _____

Phone: _____

Seizure Information:

_____
_____
_____
_____

Triggers:

_____
_____

Daily Seizure Medicine:

_____
_____
_____
_____

Feld F., Gorse KM, Blanc RO
Non-Orthopedic Emergency Care in Athletics (pp 121-123).
© 2020 Taylor & Francis Group.

Other Seizure Treatments
Device Type: _____
Model: _____
Serial#: _____
Date Implanted: _____
Dietary Therapy: _____
Date Begun: _____

Special Instructions:
_____
_____
_____
_____
_____

Other Therapy:
_____
_____
_____
_____

Seizure First Aid
  Keep calm, provide reassurance, remove bystanders
  Keep airway clear, turn on side if possible, nothing in mouth
  Keep safe, remove objects, do not restrain
  Time, observe, record what happens
  Stay with person until recovered from seizure
  Other care needed: _____

  Call 911 if . . .
  Generalized seizure longer than 5 minutes
  Two or more seizures without recovering between seizures
  "As needed" treatments do not work
  Injury occurs or is suspected or seizure occurs in water
  Breathing, heart rate, or behavior does not return to normal
  Unexplained fever or pain hours or a few days after a seizure
  Other care needed: _____

When Seizures Require Additional Help
_____
_____
_____

"As Needed" Treatments (eg, vagus nerve stimulation magnet, medicines):
_____
_____
_____
_____

Health Care Contact
Epilepsy Doctor: _____
Phone: _____
Nurse/Other Health Care Provider:_____
Phone: _____
Preferred Hospital: _____
Phone: _____
Primary Care: _____
Phone: _____
Pharmacy: _____
Phone: _____
Special Instructions: _____
_____
_____
_____

My signature: _____
Date:_____
Provider signature: _____
Date:_____

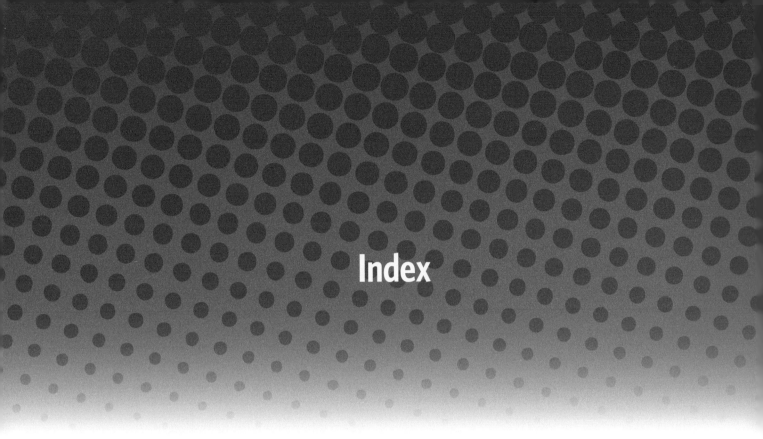

Index